Priority Areas for National Action

Transforming Health Care Quality

Karen Adams and Janet M. Corrigan, *Editors*

Committee on Identifying Priority Areas for Quality Improvement

Board on Health Care Services

INSTITUTE OF MEDICINE
OF THE NATIONAL ACADEMIES

THE NATIONAL ACADEMIES PRESS
Washington, D.C.
www.nap.edu

THE NATIONAL ACADEMIES PRESS   500 Fifth Street, N.W.   Washington, DC   20001

NOTICE: The project that is the subject of this report was approved by the Governing Board of the National Research Council, whose members are drawn from the councils of the National Academy of Sciences, the National Academy of Engineering, and the Institute of Medicine. The members of the committee responsible for the report were chosen for their special competences and with regard for appropriate balance.

Support for this project was provided by the Agency for Healthcare Research and Quality (AHRQ). The views presented in this report are those of the Institute of Medicine Committee on Identifying Priority Areas for Quality Improvement and are not necessarily those of the funding agencies.

International Standard Book Number 0-309-08543-8

Additional copies of this report are available from the National Academies Press, 500 Fifth Street, N.W., Lockbox 285, Washington, DC 20055; (800) 624-6242 or (202) 334-3313 (in the Washington metropolitan area); Internet, http://www.nap.edu.

For more information about the Institute of Medicine, visit the IOM home page at: **www.iom.edu.**

The serpent has been a symbol of long life, healing, and knowledge among almost all cultures and religions since the beginning of recorded history. The serpent adopted as a logotype by the Institute of Medicine is a relief carving from ancient Greece, now held by the Staatliche Museen in Berlin.

*"Knowing is not enough; we must apply.
Willing is not enough; we must do."*
—Goethe

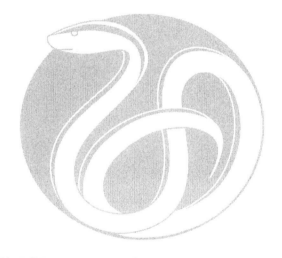

INSTITUTE OF MEDICINE

OF THE NATIONAL ACADEMIES

Shaping the Future for Health

THE NATIONAL ACADEMIES
Advisers to the Nation on Science, Engineering, and Medicine

The **National Academy of Sciences** is a private, nonprofit, self-perpetuating society of distinguished scholars engaged in scientific and engineering research, dedicated to the furtherance of science and technology and to their use for the general welfare. Upon the authority of the charter granted to it by the Congress in 1863, the Academy has a mandate that requires it to advise the federal government on scientific and technical matters. Dr. Bruce M. Alberts is president of the National Academy of Sciences.

The **National Academy of Engineering** was established in 1964, under the charter of the National Academy of Sciences, as a parallel organization of outstanding engineers. It is autonomous in its administration and in the selection of its members, sharing with the National Academy of Sciences the responsibility for advising the federal government. The National Academy of Engineering also sponsors engineering programs aimed at meeting national needs, encourages education and research, and recognizes the superior achievements of engineers. Dr. Wm. A. Wulf is president of the National Academy of Engineering.

The **Institute of Medicine** was established in 1970 by the National Academy of Sciences to secure the services of eminent members of appropriate professions in the examination of policy matters pertaining to the health of the public. The Institute acts under the responsibility given to the National Academy of Sciences by its congressional charter to be an adviser to the federal government and, upon its own initiative, to identify issues of medical care, research, and education. Dr. Harvey V. Fineberg is president of the Institute of Medicine.

The **National Research Council** was organized by the National Academy of Sciences in 1916 to associate the broad community of science and technology with the Academy's purposes of furthering knowledge and advising the federal government. Functioning in accordance with general policies determined by the Academy, the Council has become the principal operating agency of both the National Academy of Sciences and the National Academy of Engineering in providing services to the government, the public, and the scientific and engineering communities. The Council is administered jointly by both Academies and the Institute of Medicine. Dr. Bruce M. Alberts and Dr. Wm. A. Wulf are chair and vice chair, respectively, of the National Research Council.

www.national-academies.org

REVIEWERS

This report has been reviewed in draft form by individuals chosen for their diverse perspectives and technical expertise, in accordance with procedures approved by the NRC's Report Review Committee. The purpose of this independent review is to provide candid and critical comments that will assist the institution in making its published report as sound as possible and to ensure that the report meets institutional standards for objectivity, evidence, and responsiveness to the study charge. The review comments and draft manuscript remain confidential to protect the integrity of the deliberative process. We wish to thank the following individuals for their review of this report:

GERARD ANDERSON, Professor of Health Policy, Management and International Health, The Johns Hopkins School of Public Health, Baltimore, MD

LONNIE R. BRISTOW, former President, American Medical Association, Walnut Creek, CA

ADAMS DUDLEY, Assistant Professor of Medicine, Health Policy, Epidemiology and Biostatistics, Institute for Health Policy Studies, University of California San Francisco, San Francisco, CA

VALENTIN FUSTER, Director, Cardiovascular Institute and Richard Gorlin, M.D. Heart Research Foundation, Mount Sinai Medical Center, New York, NY

DAVID B. GRAY, Associate Professor of Neurology and Occupational Therapy, Washington University School of Medicine, St. Louis, MO

HURDIS M. GRIFFITH, former Dean and Professor, Rutgers, The State University of New Jersey, Arlington, VA

SAM HO, Vice President Corporate Medical Director, Pacific Health Systems, Santa Ana, CA

STEVEN E. HYMAN, Provost, Harvard University, Cambridge, MA

ELIZABETH A. MCGLYNN, The RAND Corporation, Center for Research on Quality in Health Care, Santa Monica, CA

BILL ROPER, Dean, School of Public Health, University of North Carolina at Chapel Hill, Chapel Hill, NC

ED WAGNER, Director, W.A. McColl Institute for Healthcare Innovation, Group Health Cooperative Puget Sound, Seattle, WA

Although the reviewers listed above have provided many constructive comments and suggestions, they were not asked to endorse the conclusions or recommendations nor did they see the final draft of the report before its release. The review of this report was overseen by **DONALD M. STEINWACHS**, The Johns Hopkins Bloomberg School of Public Health, Baltimore, MD and **CHARLES E. PHELPS**, University of Rochester, Rochester, NY. Appointed by the National Research Council and Institute of Medicine, they were responsible for making certain that an independent examination of this report was carried out in accordance with institutional procedures and that all review comments were carefully considered. Responsibility for the final content of this report rests entirely with the authoring committee and the institution.

Preface

In the 2001 report *Crossing the Quality Chasm: A New Health System for the 21ˢᵗ Century*, the Institute of Medicine (IOM) called for fundamental change in a troubled and ailing health care system. The change requires substantial improvements in six major aims outlined in that report – that health care be safe, effective, patient-centered, timely, efficient, and equitable. The report further suggested that the Agency for Healthcare Research and Quality (AHRQ) identify not fewer than 15 priority conditions for the purpose of developing strategies, goals, and action plans for achieving substantial improvements in quality in the next 5 years for each of the priority conditions.

In response, the Department of Health and Human Services (DHHS) contracted with the IOM to convene a committee of experts that would establish a process and a set of criteria for determining the priority conditions, identify potential candidates, and recommend to DHHS a final list of priority conditions. The committee presenting this report was constituted for that purpose. This committee was propelled forward by a short timeline for the work, as this was a "fast-track" study. The findings of this study are wanted by a number of groups that are working on projects to push transformation of the health system forward. In particular, it is envisioned that the priority areas will become subjects of AHRQ's National Health Care Quality Report. The recently released IOM report *Leadership by Example: Coordinating Government Roles in Improving Health Care Quality,* calls for the government to take the lead in promulgating standardized performance measures and points to the priority areas as the springboard for this effort. I know this committee shares a sense of urgency around the need to move forward without delay with the required re-design of the health care system.

Although chronic conditions are important candidates for quality improvement, the committee was charged and constituted to take a broader approach. The committee concluded that a purely disease based approach would not accomplish the needed transformation that the list of priority conditions intended to bring about. Thus, our scope was broader than the original focus on "priority conditions" as suggested in the *Quality Chasm* report and included other essential "priority areas" of health care, such as preventive care and behavioral health. Our list of recommended priority areas reflects this broader perspective of our task.

The committee is mindful of the dilemma presented by the fact that there are many more than the 20 areas recommended as priorities that are in need of substantial quality improvement. Nevertheless we believe that the 20 areas recommended represent a good starting point for this work because they collectively represent the full spectrum of health care from preventive and acute care to chronic disease management, to long-term and palliative care at the end of life. It is our hope that progress in quality of care in these areas will lead to changes in the underlying systems that support care and this progress will also benefit those with many conditions that are not included in this first list of recommended priority areas.

I am grateful to have had the opportunity to work with a dedicated, talented and energetic committee on this project. We were well supported by Karen Adams, program officer and Danitza Valdivia, project assistant both staff of the IOM. The generous insights of our workshop presenters and those members of the public giving testimony and communication assisted us in great measure.

With these priority areas as a starting point, it's now time to get on with the implementation of changes that are necessary to transform our health care system into something of which we can truly be proud.

George Isham, M.D., M.S.
Chair
January 2003

Foreword

This report is one in a series spearheaded by the Institute of Medicine (IOM) to improve the quality of health care in America. The IOM's quality initiative has gone through three stages since its genesis 6 years ago. In its first phase, the National Roundtable on Health Care Quality, convened by the IOM, highlighted serious problems in the quality of care and noted them to be pervasive throughout the country. The work of this group heightened awareness of the overuse, misuse, and underuse of health care services that harm large numbers of Americans every day. The second phase of our quality initiative, from 1999-2001, was marked by the release of two reports *To Err is Human* and *Crossing the Quality Chasm,* both of which called for drastic redesign of our health care delivery system to narrow the gap between the best clinical practice and the usual practice today.

We are now fully immersed in phase three of our quality initiative and have begun to lay the groundwork for implementing the recommendations set forth in *Crossing the Quality Chasm.* This report responds to the call in *Crossing the Quality Chasm,* for a limited set of priority areas, predominately chronic conditions, which would serve as the starting point for restructuring our health care delivery system. It was envisioned that stakeholders from health care organizations, purchasers, professional groups, and most importantly, consumers would join forces and take action to improve quality in these select areas within the next five years.

The majority of priority areas recommended in this report are chronic conditions; however, the final list also represents the many realms of health care, including preventive care, acute care, and end of life care. Many of the priority areas targeted are the leading causes of death in the United States. Their toll on human life is great. Behind each of these priority areas are many individuals who are not receiving optimal care. Each of these priority areas can be a locus to transform our health care system into one that is more fully integrated and responsive to patient needs. This will require the collective efforts of organizations and individuals, many of which have already begun hard work in these areas. In addition to restructuring how care is delivered, the priority areas can also be the warp to weave information technology into the fabric of daily clinical decision-making and set the stage for linking payment incentives to the quality of care. These priority areas are thus important in their own rights and as focal points to improve the quality of health care.

Harvey Fineberg, M.D., PhD
President, Institute of Medicine
January 2003

Acknowledgments

The Committee on Identifying Priority Areas for Quality Improvement wishes to acknowledge the many people whose contributions made this report possible. We appreciate how willingly and generously these individuals contributed their time and expertise to assist the committee with their deliberations.

The following individuals participated in a workshop panel or addressed the committee: Gerard Anderson, the Johns Hopkins School of Public Health; Brian Austin, Macoll Institute for Healthcare Innovation; Dan Brock, Brown University; Carolyn Clancy, Agency for Healthcare Research and Quality; Ashley Coffield, Partnership for Prevention; Steve Cohen, Agency for Healthcare Research and Quality; Helen Darling, Washington Business Group on Health; Suzanne Delbanco, Leapfrog Group; Benjamin Druss, Yale School of Medicine; Charlene Harrington, University of California, San Francisco; Brent James, Intermountain Health Care; Bob Kafka, American Disabled for Accessible Public Transit; Joanne Lynn, Americans for Better Care of the Dying; Michael Maciosek, HealthPartners; Ali Mokdad, Centers for Disease Control and Prevention; James Perrin, Harvard Medical School; Kip Piper, National Healthcare Purchasing Institute; Nico Pronk, HealthPartners; David Stevens, Health Resources and Services Administration; Mary Tinetti, Yale School of Medicine; and Kenneth Wells, University of California, Los Angeles.

Other individuals who made important contributions to the committee's work: Karen Beauregard, Steve Cohen and Nancy Kraus from the Agency for Healthcare Research and Quality, who provided technical assistance with MEPS survey data.

Support for this project was provided by the Agency for Healthcare Research and Quality.

Contents

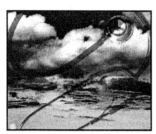# Executive Summary

This report follows several studies spearheaded by the Institute of Medicine (IOM) and other groups that document disturbing shortfalls in the quality of health care in the United States. The following statement prepared for the National Roundtable on Health Care Quality captures the magnitude and scope of the problem:

> Serious and widespread quality problems exist throughout American medicine....[They] occur in small and large communities alike, in all parts of the country and with approximately equal frequency in managed care and fee-for-service systems of care. Very large numbers of Americans are harmed as a result (Chassin and Galvin, 1998:1000).

Likewise, two subsequent IOM studies—*To Err is Human: Building a Safer Health System* (Institute of Medicine, 2000) and *Crossing the Quality Chasm: A New Health System for the 21st Century* (Institute of Medicine, 2001a)—focus national attention on patient safety concerns surrounding the high incidence of medical errors and sizable gaps in health care quality, respectively.

In addition to the IOM, many others have assumed leadership roles in the movement to address and improve health care safety and quality. These efforts have included both large-scale national initiatives, such as the President's Advisory Commission on Consumer Protection and Quality in the Health Care Industry (1998) and Healthy People 2010 (United States Department of Health and Human Services, 2000), and private efforts such as the work of the RAND Corporation, which resulted in a call for mandatory tracking and reporting of health care quality (Schuster et al., 1998). The newly released chart book from the Commonwealth Fund, which examines the current status of quality of health care in the United States, confirms that quality problems persist (Leatherman and McCarthy, 2002):

- Fewer than half of adults aged 50 and over were found to have received recommended screening tests for colorectal cancer (Centers for Disease Control and Prevention, 2001; Leatherman and McCarthy, 2002).

- Inadequate care after a heart attack results in 18,000 unnecessary deaths per year (Chassin, 1997).

- In a recent survey, 17 million people reported being told by their pharmacist that the drugs they were prescribed could cause an interaction (Harris Interactive, 2001).

Problems such as those cited above have now been noted so frequently that we risk becoming desensitized even as we pursue change. Our technical lexicon of performance improvements and system interventions can obscure the stark reality that we invest billions in research to find appropriate treatments (National Institutes of Health, 2002), we spend more than $1 trillion on health care annually (Heffler et al., 2002), we have extraordinary knowledge and capacity to deliver the best care in the world, but we repeatedly fail to translate that knowledge and capacity into clinical practice.

Study Purpose and Scope

The IOM's *Quality Chasm* report sets forth a bold strategy for achieving substantial improvement in health care quality during the coming decade (Institute of Medicine, 2001a). As a crucial first step in making the nation's health care system more responsive to the needs of patients and more capable of delivering science-based care, the *Quality Chasm* report recommends the systematic identification of priority areas for quality improvement. The idea behind this strategy was to have various groups at different levels focus on improving care in a limited set of priority areas, with the hope that their collective efforts would help move the nation forward toward achieving

better-quality health care for all Americans. In response, the Department of Health and Human Services (DHHS) contracted with the IOM to form a committee whose charge was threefold: to select criteria for screening potential priority areas, to develop a process for applying those criteria, and to generate a list of approximately 15 to 20 candidate areas.

Guiding Principles

Systems Approach

Behind each of the priority areas recommended in this report is a patient who may be receiving poor quality care. This is due not to a lack of effective treatments, but to inadequate health care delivery systems that fail to implement these treatments. For this reason, the committee considered quality to be a systems property, recognizing that although the health care workforce is trying hard to deliver the best care, those efforts are doomed to failure with today's outmoded and poorly designed systems. The committee did not concentrate on ways of improving the efficacy of existing best-practice treatments through either biomedical research or technological innovation, but rather on ways to improve the delivery of those treatments. Indeed the goal of the study was to identify priority areas that presented the greatest opportunity to narrow the gap between what the health care system is routinely doing now and what we know to be best medical practice.

Scope and Framework

The *Quality Chasm* report proposes that chronic conditions serve as the focal point for the priority areas, given that a limited number of chronic conditions account for the majority of the nation's health care burden and resource use (Hoffman et al., 1996; Institute of Medicine, 2001a; Partnership for Solutions, 2001; The Robert Wood Johnson Foundation, 2001). Chronic conditions do represent a substantial number of the priority areas on the final list presented in this report; however, this committee was constituted and charged to go beyond a disease-based approach. Therefore, the committee decided to recommend priority areas that would be representative of the entire spectrum of health care, rather than being limited to one important segment.

Given this broader perspective, the committee decided a framework would be useful in helping to identify potential candidates for the priority areas. The committee built upon the framework originally developed by the Foundation for Accountability and subsequently incorporated into the National Health Care Quality Report (Foundation for Accountability, 1997a, 1997b; Institute of Medicine, 2001b). This consumer-oriented framework encompasses four domains of care: staying healthy (preventive care), getting better (acute care), living with illness/disability (chronic care), and coping with end of life (palliative care).[1] In response to the *Quality Chasm* report's ardent appeal for systems change, the committee supplemented these four categories with a fifth—cross-cutting systems interventions—to address vitally important areas, such as coordination of care, that cut across specific conditions and domains.

Like all frameworks, that employed by the committee has advantages as well as limitations. The committee found its framework to be useful for initially identifying candidate areas and then later in the process for checking the balance of the final portfolio of recommended priority areas. However, one of the framework's limitations was that it tended to result in placing conditions into rigid categories, whereas health care for many of the priority areas involves services in all five categories. Figure ES-1 presents the committee's initial framework for determining priority areas. The overlapping circles represent the interrelatedness of the five categories.

Recommendation 1: The committee recommends that the priority areas collectively:

- **Represent the U.S. population's health care needs across the lifespan, in multiple health care settings involving many types of health care professionals.**

- **Extend across the full spectrum of health care, from keeping people well and maximizing overall health; to providing treatment to cure people of disease and health problems as often as possible; to assisting people who become chronically ill to live longer, more productive and comfortable lives; to providing dignified care at the end of life that is respectful of the values and preferences of individuals and their families.**

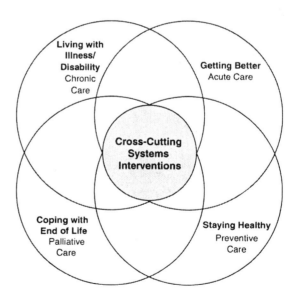

FIGURE ES-1 The committee's initial framework for determining priority areas.

---

[1] Terms in parentheses are the clinical terms corresponding to each of these stages.

Evidence-Based Approach

The committee developed its recommendations using an evidence-based approach. Particularly for estimates of disease burden, the committee relied on quantitative data from national datasets to compare the burden of disease as regards prevalence, disability, and costs across priority areas.

At the same time, the committee recognized that the existing evidence base could provide only partial guidance for fulfilling its charge. Specifically, there was little quantitative data available for comparing the costs and outcomes of quality improvement programs across different priority areas. For this purpose, the committee supplemented quantitative data with qualitative data and case studies of successful examples of system change. These sources were used to study whether, for a condition posing a high health burden, there was evidence that quality improvement could substantially improve care. Here, the committee used evidence to examine the potential benefits of system change, rather than to generate numerical rankings for particular priority areas. To ensure a stronger evidence base in the future, the committee has recommended strategic investment in research on effective interventions that can improve the quality of care in a number of the priority areas and the development of accompanying standardized measures.

Criteria

The committee used three closely related criteria—impact, improvability, and inclusiveness—in selecting the priority areas.

Recommendation 2: The committee recommends use of the following criteria for identifying priority areas:

- *Impact*—**the extent of the burden—disability, mortality, and economic costs—imposed by a condition, including effects on patients, families, communities, and societies.**

- *Improvability*—**the extent of the gap between current practice and evidence-based best practice and the likelihood that the gap can be closed and conditions improved through change in an area; and the opportunity to achieve dramatic improvements in the six national quality aims identified in the *Quality Chasm* report (safety, effectiveness, patient-centeredness, timeliness, efficiency and equity).**

- *Inclusiveness*—**the relevance of an area to a broad range of individuals with regard to age, gender, socioeconomic status, and ethnicity/ race (equity); the generalizability of associated quality improvement strategies to many types of conditions and illnesses across the spectrum of health care (representativeness); and the breadth of change effected through such strategies across a range of health care settings and providers (reach).**

Final List of Priority Areas

The committee's selection process yielded a final set of 20 priority areas for improvement in health care quality. Improving the delivery of care in any of these areas would enable stakeholders at the national, state, and local levels to begin setting a course for quality health care while addressing unacceptable disparities in care for all Americans. The committee made no attempt to rank order the priority areas selected. The first 2 listed—care coordination and self-management/health literacy—are cross-cutting areas in which improvements would benefit a broad array of patients. The 17 that follow represent the continuum of care across the life span and are relevant to preventive care, inpatient/surgical care, chronic conditions, end-of-life care, and behavioral health, as well as to care for children and adolescents (see boxes ES-1 to ES-6). Finally, obesity is included as an "emerging area"[2] that does not at this point satisfy the selection criteria as fully as the other 19 priority areas.

Recommendation 3: The committee recommends that DHHS, along with other public and private entities, focus on the following priority areas for transforming health care:

- **Care coordination (cross-cutting)**
- **Self-management/health literacy (cross-cutting)**
- **Asthma—appropriate treatment for persons with mild/moderate persistent asthma**
- **Cancer screening that is evidence-based—focus on colorectal and cervical cancer**
- **Children with special health care needs** [3]

- **Diabetes—focus on appropriate management of early disease**
- **End of life with advanced organ system failure—focus on congestive heart failure and chronic obstructive pulmonary disease**
- **Frailty associated with old age—preventing falls and pressure ulcers, maximizing function, and developing advanced care plans**
- **Hypertension—focus on appropriate management of early disease**
- **Immunization—children and adults**
- **Ischemic heart disease—prevention, reduction of recurring events, and optimization of functional capacity**
- **Major depression—screening and treatment**
- **Medication management—preventing medication errors and overuse of antibiotics**
- **Nosocomial infections—prevention and surveillance**
- **Pain control in advanced cancer**
- **Pregnancy and childbirth—appropriate prenatal and intrapartum care**
- **Severe and persistent mental illness—focus on treatment in the public sector**
- **Stroke—early intervention and rehabilitation**
- **Tobacco dependence treatment in adults**
- **Obesity (emerging area)**

---

[2] An emerging area is one of high burden (impact) that affects a broad range of individuals (inclusiveness) and for which the evidence base for effective interventions (improvability) is still forming.

[3] The Maternal and Child Health Bureau defines this population as "those (children) who have or are at increased risk for a chronic physical, developmental, behavioral or emotional condition and who also require health and related services of a type or amount beyond that required by children generally" (McPherson et al., 1998:138).

Box ES-1 Priority Areas That Relate to Preventive Care

- Care coordination (cross-cutting)
- Self-management/health literacy (cross-cutting)
- Cancer screening
- Hypertension
- Immunization
- Ischemic heart disease (prevention)
- Major depression (screening)
- Pregnancy and childbirth
- Tobacco dependence
- Obesity (emerging area)

Box ES-2 Priority Areas That Relate to Behavioral Health

- Care coordination (cross-cutting)
- Self-management/health literacy (cross-cutting)
- Major depression
- Severe and persistent mental illness
- Tobacco dependence
- Obesity (emerging area)

Box ES-3 Priority Areas That Relate to Chronic Conditions

- Care coordination (cross-cutting)
- Self-management/health literacy (cross-cutting)
- Asthma
- Children with special health care needs
- Diabetes
- End of life with advanced organ system failure
- Frailty
- Hypertension
- Ischemic heart disease
- Major depression (treatment)
- Medication management
  - Medication errors
  - Overuse of antibiotics
- Pain control in advanced cancer
- Severe and persistent mental illness
- Stroke
- Tobacco dependence
- Obesity (emerging area)

Box ES-4 Priority Areas That Relate to End of Life

- Care coordination (cross-cutting)
- Self-management/health literacy (cross-cutting)
- Chronic conditions
- End of life with advanced organ system failure
- Frailty
- Medication management
  - Medication errors
  - Overuse of antibiotics
- Nosocomial infections
- Pain control in advanced cancer

Box ES-5 Priority Areas That Relate to Children and Adolescents

- Care coordination (cross-cutting)
- Self-management/health literacy (cross-cutting)
- Asthma
- Children with special health care needs
- Diabetes
- Immunization (children)
- Major depression
- Medication management
  - Medication errors
  - Overuse of antibiotics
- Obesity (emerging area)

Box ES-6 Priority Areas That Relate to Inpatient/Surgical Care

- Care coordination (cross-cutting)
- Self-management/health literacy (cross-cutting)
- End of life with advanced organ system failure
- Ischemic heart disease
- Medication management
  - Medication errors
  - Overuse of antibiotics
- Nosocomial infections
- Pain control in advanced cancer
- Pregnancy and childbirth
- Severe and persistent mental illness
- Stroke

Process for Identifying Priority Areas

In response to its charge, the committee developed a process for determining priority areas (see Figure ES-2). This process was refined according to the committee's experience in selecting the priority areas recommended in this report, and is suggested as a model for future priority-setting efforts. The steps in the process can be summarized as follows:

1. Determine a framework for the priority areas.

2. Identify candidate areas.

3. Establish criteria for selecting the final priority areas.

4. Categorize candidate areas within the framework.

5. Apply impact and inclusiveness criteria to the candidates.

6. Apply criteria of improvability and inclusiveness to the preliminary set of areas obtained in step 5.

7. Identify priority areas; reassess and approve.

8. Implement strategies for improving care in the priority areas, measure the impact of implementation, and review/update the list of areas.

Throughout the process, public input should be solicited from multiple sources.

Following is a detailed description of each of the above steps. This description encompasses both the process initially formulated by the committee and modifications that emerged as a result of the committee's deliberations.

Determine Framework

The framework used by the committee's was discussed above and is detailed in Chapter 1.

Identify Candidates

In developing an initial candidate list, the committee drew on a variety of sources. These included the collective knowledge and broad expertise of its members (see Appendix A for biographical sketches of committee members), feedback received from presenters and the public at a workshop held in May 2002 (see Appendix B for the workshop agenda), and work done by other groups in the area of the burden of chronic conditions/diseases and by organizations that have already established lists of priority conditions/areas to meet their specific needs. Using all these resources, the committee settled on a list of approximately 60 candidate priority areas to screen by means of the process outlined above. Selecting just 60 candidates for the first cut was extremely difficult, as there are hundreds of diseases, preventive services, and health care system failures that might be included. The remaining steps in the process were then applied to narrow this list still further to the 20 areas recommended by the committee.

Establish Criteria

The criteria used by the committee were cited above and are discussed in depth in Chapter 2.

Categorize Candidates Within the Framework

Once a pool of candidate areas had been established, they were organized within the categories of the framework. For example, using the committee's initial framework, diabetes was placed under chronic care, tobacco dependency treatment under preventive care, pain control under palliative care, antibiotic overuse under acute care, and care coordination under cross-cutting systems interventions.

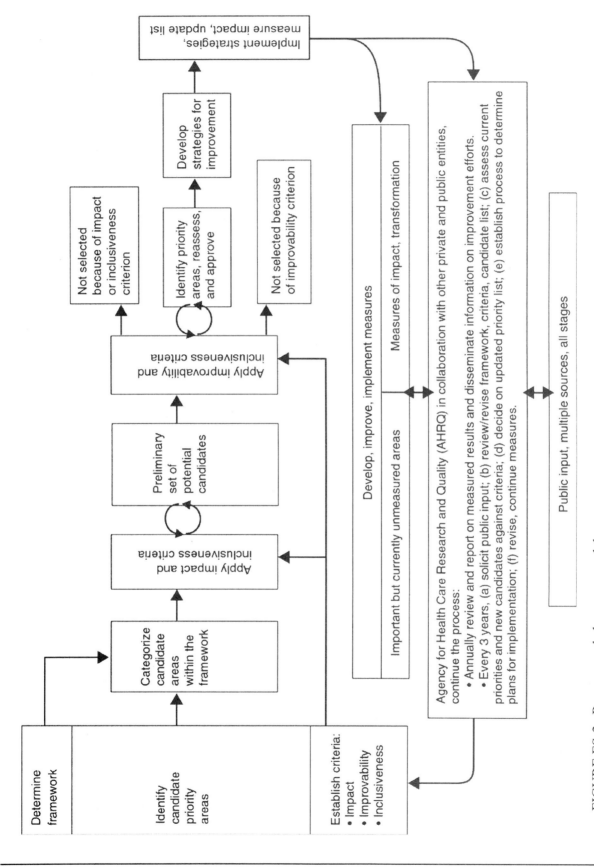

FIGURE ES-2 Recommended process model.

Apply Criteria to Candidates

After identifying a list of candidate priority areas and organizing them within the framework, the committee applied the selection criteria to each area, being particularly sensitive to the impact on disadvantaged populations. All three criteria were applied in a single step when the committee performed this selection process. On the basis of its experience, however, the committee recommends a two-step process for future efforts: one should screen for impact first, then for improvability, and throughout the process, particular attention should be paid to inclusiveness. This two-step approach would identify more clearly for consumers, practitioners, and researchers the rationale for including some areas and not others. It would elucidate, for example, which areas did not meet the impact criterion and which met this criterion but not that of improvability. Such clarification could help shape future work in the areas involved. Moreover, future applications of this approach to update the priority areas might well involve richer data analysis and more extensive feedback from the public and health professionals.

Identify Priority Areas

The priority areas selected by the committee were listed earlier under recommendation 3 and are discussed in more detail in Chapter 3.

Next Steps

With the priority areas having been identified, the final step in the process is to implement strategies for improving care in the priority areas, measure the impact of implementation, and periodically review/update the list of areas. Impact should be measured using methods that are standardized and can permit comparison across these diverse areas of quality improvement. The assessment must include measures of the degree to which the system has been transformed and of the clinical impact on patient care. As such changes are effected, the list of priority areas should be reviewed and updated—optimally every 3 to 5 years. Other areas may need to be added to the list as the result of new data on impact or the development of new treatment interventions. Likewise, if strategies for improvement are effective, it may be possible to remove some areas from the list.

Recommendation 4: The committee recommends that the Agency for Healthcare Research and Quality (AHRQ), in collaboration with other private and public organizations, be responsible for continuous assessment of progress and updating of the list of priority areas. These responsibilities should include:

- **Developing and improving data collection and measurement systems for assessing the effectiveness of quality improvement efforts.**

- **Supporting the development and dissemination of valid, accurate, and reliable standardized measures of quality.**

- **Measuring key attributes and outcomes and making this information available to the public.**

- **Revising the selection criteria and the list of priority areas.**

- **Reviewing the evidence base and results, and deciding on updated priorities every 3 to 5 years.**

- **Assessing changes in the attributes of society that affect health and health care and could alter the priority of various areas.**

- **Disseminating the results of strategies for quality improvement in the priority areas.**

Throughout this study, the committee often encountered a lack of reliable measures to use in assessing improvability for the priority areas under consideration. Available datasets, although useful, were also limited in that they were unable to provide information on health status and health functioning because of their disease - and procedure-based orientation. In addition, it was difficult to compare many quality improvement efforts because of a lack of standardization in the way outcomes were measured. Thus, the committee concluded that particular attention should be focused on enhancing survey data and developing new strategies for collecting, collating, and disseminating quality improvement data. Those conducting quality improvement studies should be encouraged to include a core set of measures that would allow comparability across different conditions, just as consensus standards have been developed for conducting and reporting cost-effectiveness analyses (Gold, 1996; Russell et al., 1996; Siegel et al., 1996; Weinstein et al., 1996). Only with such standardized approaches will it be possible to use findings from quality improvement studies for future efforts at priority setting.

Recommendation 5: The committee recommends that data collection in the priority areas:

- **Go beyond the usual reliance on disease - and procedure-based information to include data on the health and functioning of the U.S. population.**

- **Cover relevant demographic and regional groups, as well as the population as a whole, with particular emphasis on identifying disparities in care.**

- **Be consistent within and across categories to ensure accurate assessment and comparison of quality enhancement efforts.**

If AHRQ is to spearhead this undertaking, appropriate funds must be allocated for the purpose. National experts should be convened to develop action plans in the priority areas, and this should be done expeditiously so as to sustain momentum and ensure the timeliness of the committee's recommendations.

Recommendation 6: The committee recommends that the Congress and the Administration provide the necessary support for the ongoing process of monitoring progress in the priority areas and updating the list of areas. This support should encompass:

- **The administrative costs borne by AHRQ.**

- **The costs of developing and implementing data collection mechanisms and improving the capacity to measure results.**

- **The costs of investing strategically in research aimed at developing new scientific evidence on interventions that improve the quality of care and at creating additional accurate, valid, and reliable standardized measures of quality. Such research is especially critical in areas of high importance in which either the scientific evidence for effective interventions is lacking, or current measures of quality are inadequate.**

The list of priority areas identified by the committee is intended to serve as a starting point for transforming the nation's health care system. Many of the leading causes of death are on this list. Just five of the conditions included—heart disease, cancer, stroke, chronic obstructive pulmonary disease, and diabetes—account for approximately 1.5 million deaths annually and represent 63 percent of total deaths in the United States (Minino and Smith, 2001).[4] If redesigning systems of care resulted in merely a 5 percent mortality improvement in these areas alone, nearly 75,000 premature deaths could potentially be averted.

Although AHRQ's role in monitoring progress and updating the list of areas will be

---

[4] Heart disease (ischemic heart disease and hypertension), 537,088; cancer, 551,833; stroke, 166,028; chronic obstructive pulmonary disease, 123,550; diabetes, 68,662. Total = 1,447,161; total deaths all causes = 2,404,598.

critical, the health care system will be changed only through the individual and organized actions of patients, families, doctors, nurses, other health professionals, and administrators; no national body or collaboration can accomplish the task alone. The priority areas deliberately encompass a wide range of health care issues in which improvement is needed for overall system change. However, the priorities are also specific enough that individuals and organizations can choose areas on which to focus their improvement efforts, helping to guarantee that all Americans will receive the quality health care they deserve.

References

Centers for Disease Control and Prevention. 2001. Trends in screening for colorectal cancer—United States, 1997 and 1999. *Morbidity and Mortality Weekly Report* 50:161-66.

Chassin, M. R. 1997. Assessing strategies for quality improvement. *Health Aff (Millwood)* 16 (3):151-61.

Chassin, M. R., and R. W. Galvin. 1998. The urgent need to improve health care quality. Institute of Medicine National Roundtable on Health Care Quality. *JAMA* 280 (11):1000-5.

Foundation for Accountability. 1997a. "The FACCT Consumer Information Framework: Comparative Information for Better Health Care Decisions." Online. Available at http://www.facct.org/information.html [accessed June 4, 2002].

———. 1997b. *Reporting Quality Information to Consumers*. Portland, OR: FACCT.

Gold, M. R. 1996. *Cost-effectiveness in health and medicine*. New York: Oxford University Press.

Harris Interactive. 2001. *Survey on Chronic Illness and Caregiving*. New York: Harris Interactive.

Heffler, S., S. Smith, G. Won, M. K. Clemens, S. Keehan, and M. Zezza. 2002. Health spending projections for 2001-2011: The latest outlook. Faster health spending growth and a slowing economy drive the health spending projection for 2001 up sharply. *Health Aff (Millwood)* 21 (2):207-18.

Hoffman, C., D. Rice, and H. Y. Sung. 1996. Persons with chronic conditions: Their prevalence and costs. *JAMA* 276 (18):1473-9.

Institute of Medicine. 2000. *To Err Is Human: Building a Safer Health System.* L. T. Kohn, J. M. Corrigan, and M. S. Donaldson, eds. Washington, D.C: National Academy Press.

———. 2001a. *Crossing the Quality Chasm: A New Health System for the 21st Century.* Washington, D.C.: National Academy Press.

———. 2001b. *Envisioning the National Health Care Quality Report.* M. P. Hurtado, E. K. Swift, and J. M. Corrigan, eds. Washington, D.C.: National Academy Press.

Leatherman, S. and D. McCarthy. 2002. *Quality of Health Care in the United States: A Chartbook*. New York, NY: The Commonwealth Fund.

McPherson, M., P. Arango, H. Fox, C. Lauver, M. McManus, P. W. Newacheck, J. M. Perrin, J. P. Shonkoff, and B. Strickland. 1998. A new definition of children with special health care needs. *Pediatrics* 102 (1 Pt 1):137-40.

Minino, A. M. and B. L. Smith. 2001. *National Vital Statistics Reports*. Centers for Disease Control and Prevention.

National Institutes of Health. 2002. "NIH Press Release for the FY 2003 President's Budget." Online. Available at www.nih.gov/news/budgetfy2003/2003NIHpresbudget.htm [accessed Aug. 8, 2002].

Partnership for Solutions, The Johns Hopkins University. 2001. "Partnership for Solutions: A National Program of The Robert Wood Johnson Foundation." Online. Available at http://www.partnershipforsolutions.org/statistics/prevalence.htm [accessed Dec. 12, 2002].

President's Advisory Commission on Consumer Protection and Quality in the Health Care Industry. 1998. *Quality First: Better Health Care for All Americans—Final Report to the President of the United States*. Washington, D.C.: U.S. Government Printing Office.

Russell, L. B., M. R. Gold, J. E. Siegel, N. Daniels, and M. C. Weinstein. 1996. The role of cost-effectiveness analysis in health and medicine. Panel on Cost-Effectiveness in Health and Medicine. *JAMA* 276 (14):1172-7.

Schuster, M. A., E. A. McGlynn, and R. H. Brook. 1998. How good is the quality of health care in the United States? *Milbank Q* 76 (4):517-63, 509.

Siegel, J. E., M. C. Weinstein, L. B. Russell, and M. R. Gold. 1996. Recommendations for reporting cost-effectiveness analyses. Panel on Cost-Effectiveness in Health and Medicine. *JAMA* 276 (16):1339-41.

The Robert Wood Johnson Foundation. 2001. *A Portrait of the Chronically Ill in America.* Princeton, NJ: Robert Wood Johnson Foundation.

United States Department of Health and Human Services. 2000. *Healthy People 2010: Understanding and Improving Health.* 2nd edition. Washington, D.C.: U.S. Government Printing Office.

Weinstein, M. C., J. E. Siegel, M. R. Gold, M. S. Kamlet, and L. B. Russell. 1996. Recommendations of the Panel on Cost-effectiveness in Health and Medicine. *JAMA* 276 (15):1253-8.

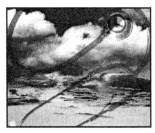

Chapter One
Introduction

In recent years, numerous reports have called attention to serious and widespread problems in the quality of health care provided to Americans. In 1998, a statement prepared for the National Roundtable on Health Care Quality asserts that many patients are harmed unnecessarily by the care they receive and that quality problems are not limited to any particular geographic area or type of health plan, whether managed care or fee-for-service (Chassin and Galvin, 1998). Likewise, a 1999 report of the IOM's National Cancer Policy Board reveals that many individuals with cancer do not receive care known to be effective for their conditions (Institute of Medicine, 1999). A subsequent report by the IOM's Committee on the Quality of Health Care in America, *To Err Is Human: Building a Safer Health System*, focused national attention on problems in patient safety and the need to design safer care processes and systems (Institute of Medicine, 2000).

The IOM is not alone in calling attention to health care safety and quality concerns. Almost 30 years ago, geographic variations in the delivery of health care were observed (Wennberg and Gittelsohn, 1973) and these variations persist today (Chassin et al., 1987; O'Connor et al., 1999; Welch et al., 1993). In 1998, the President's Advisory Commission on Consumer Protection and Quality in the Health Care Industry offered major recommendations for improving the quality of care for Americans. These recommendations included establishing public–private partnerships to provide national leadership in health care quality improvement, promoting the measurement and reporting of the quality of care delivered, and investing in information technology infrastructure to support decision making and the delivery of quality care (President's Advisory Commission on Consumer Protection and Quality in the Health Care Industry, 1998). A literature review published by the RAND Corporation in 1998 also calls for routine, mandatory tracking and reporting on the quality of care delivered to the American people (Schuster et al., 1998). And the Commonwealth Fund's newly released *Quality of Health Care in the United States: A Chartbook* confirms that large gaps persist between the care patients should and actually do receive (Leatherman and McCarthy, 2002):

- Poor treatment of diabetes result in tens of thousands of cases of premature death, limb amputation, kidney disease and blindness (American Diabetes Association, 2002; Centers for Disease Control and Prevention, 2002).

- Inadequate care after a heart attack results in 18,000 unnecessary deaths per year (Chassin, 1997).

- The average Medicare beneficiary having one or more chronic conditions is seen by eight different physicians during a year (Anderson and Knickman, 2001). Results of a recent survey indicate that approximately 20 million Americans with chronic illnesses received contradictory information from different health care providers, and 17 million reported being told by their pharmacist that the drugs they were prescribed could have interactions (Harris Interactive, 2001).

- Fewer than half of adults aged 50 and over were found to have received recommended screening tests for colorectal cancer, the second most common cause of cancer death in the United States (Centers for Disease Control and Prevention, 2001; Leatherman and McCarthy, 2002).

The 2001 IOM report *Crossing the Quality Chasm: A New Health System for the 21st Century* sets forth an ambitious agenda for taking the first steps in redesigning how health care is routinely delivered (Institute of Medicine, 2001a). The report recommends focusing greater attention on the development of care processes for common chronic conditions. The rationale for this emphasis is that targeting those conditions that account for the majority of health care burden and expenditures and making real changes in the care delivery processes for those conditions would benefit a sizable portion of the population. Moreover, a focus on enhancing quality for a few well-selected priority conditions would be likely to generate

systems, skills, awareness, and a culture that would foster improvements in other areas as well. In addition, since many conditions are treated in more than one health care setting, a focus on priority conditions might be expected to encompass care provided in physicians' offices, hospitals, and nursing homes, as well as home care settings. The *Quality Chasm* report therefore recommends that the Agency for Healthcare Research and Quality (AHRQ) within the Department of Health and Human Services (DHHS) identify no fewer than 15 priority conditions that might serve as the starting point for transforming the delivery of health care (Institute of Medicine, 2001a).

In response, DHHS contracted with the IOM to convene a committee of experts that would establish a process and develop a set of criteria for determining the priority conditions, identify candidate conditions, and recommend to DHHS a final list of priority conditions deserving of immediate attention. The IOM established a committee with broad-based representation from the following areas: public health, prevention, medicine, nursing, chronic disease management, behavioral medicine, epidemiology, quality of care, health care delivery/policy, health economics, consumer groups, geriatrics, mental health, and special populations (see Appendix A for biographies of the committee members). This report presents the results of the committee's efforts.

The next step will be to work with various stakeholders in the health care community to develop and implement strategies for improving the quality of care for each priority condition within the next 5 years. To encourage action by other stakeholders, DHSS intends to review the committee's recommendations; select priorities; and begin incorporating them into the National Health Care Quality Report, to be released for the first time in 2003 (Institute of Medicine, 2001b). That congressionally mandated report is intended to track the progress of the six national quality aims delineated in the *Quality Chasm* report: safety, effectiveness, patient-centeredness, timeliness, efficiency, and equity (Institute of Medicine, 2001a).

Study Approach

The committee developed its recommendations using an evidence-based approach whenever possible. While such evidence is essential, however, it cannot do justice to the avoidable harm that occurs in the current health care system. The priority areas recommended in this report encompass conditions for which patients are often receiving substandard care. This poor-quality care is due not to a lack of effective treatments, but to disjointed health care delivery systems that are unable to put these treatments into practice. Hence, the committee's focus was on identifying the greatest opportunities for closing the gap between known best practice and usual practice and for reducing unwarranted variation in practice, with an emphasis on changes that must be made in the health care system to exploit those opportunities. The committee also dealt with quality as a systems property—not just the responsibility of overtaxed health care workers, but flowing naturally from the improved structure of redesigned systems of care.

The committee's charge did not encompass evaluating the prospects for improving existing best-practice treatments through biomedical research or technological innovations. Rather, the committee focused on means of enhancing the delivery of those treatments. As affirmed in the *Quality Chasm* report (Institute of Medicine, 2001a:4): "The current care systems cannot do the job. Trying harder will not work. Changing systems of care will." Improving the delivery of care in the 20 specific priority areas recommended by the committee by changing systems of care would provide a way for stakeholders at the national, state, and local levels to begin setting the course toward quality health care, along with reducing unacceptable disparities among Americans (Institute of Medicine, 2002a; Institute of Medicine, 2002c).

This study was designed as a "fast-track" effort. The committee met three times over a 3-month period. A public workshop also was held to provide an opportunity for the committee to hear from experts in the areas of mental health, child/adolescent health, long-term care, disability, end of life, and preventive care and to receive input from special-interest groups, the business community, and others (see Appendix B for the workshop agenda). Between meetings, the committee also made extensive use of subgroups. Immediately following the first meeting, three subgroups were formed to refine a set of preliminary criteria for the selection of priority areas, to craft a process for identifying the priority areas in a systematic and thoughtful manner, and to examine measurement issues involved in determining the final list of areas. Between the second and third meetings, two subgroups were formed to filter the initial slate of priority areas through a process agreed upon by the committee. The third and final meeting was spent deliberating the priority areas and formulating recommendations for this report.

It was originally envisioned that the priority areas would consist of common clinical conditions, most of which would be chronic in nature (Institute of Medicine, 2001a). The charge from AHRQ to the committee reflected this view. For several decades, the health care needs of the American people have been shifting from predominately acute care to chronic care. Today, chronic conditions are the leading cause of illness, disability, and death in the United States. In the year 2000, nearly half of the U.S. population, or approximately 125 million people, had such a condition. This figure is projected to increase to 157 million by 2020. In addition, 60 million Americans have two or more chronic conditions. Such chronic conditions also account for the majority of health care expenditures. In the year 2000, the direct costs of care for chronic conditions totaled $510 billion, and this figure is estimated to double to $1.07 trillion by 2020 (Partnership for Solutions, 2001).

The nation's health care delivery systems have not significantly evolved to meet these changing demands. It has become increasingly clear that existing health care systems are designed to provide acute and emergency care and must be redesigned to deliver the type of planned, proactive care needed to prevent and manage chronic disease. Although some patients receive well-orchestrated quality care, far too many others must navigate through a tangled web of health professionals and medical facilities. The result is often profound frustration and confusion on behalf of patients, families, and health care providers, which in turn increases the risk that health care needs will not be adequately met and contributes to disparities in care among social, ethnic, and socioeconomic groups (Anderson and Knickman, 2001; Hoffman et al., 1996; Institute of Medicine, 2002c; Wagner et al., 1996).

Although chronic conditions are clearly central candidates for quality improvement, the committee was charged and purposely constituted to adopt a more comprehensive approach. Thus, the scope of the study was broadened from the original focus on "priority conditions" as suggested in the *Quality Chasm*

report to include other essential "priority areas" of health care, such as preventive care and behavioral health. Indeed, one of the committee's main conclusions was that a purely disease-based approach to health care would not accomplish the needed transformation that is the intent of the recommended list of priority areas.

The committee decided a framework would be useful in the initial identification of candidate priority areas. Consistent with its charge, it built upon a framework originally formulated by the Foundation for Accountability that is to be incorporated into the National Health Care Quality Report (Foundation for Accountability, 1997a; 1997b; Institute of Medicine, 2001b). This consumer-oriented framework encompasses four domains of care: staying healthy (preventive care), getting better (acute care), living with illness/disability (chronic care), and coping with end of life (palliative care).[1] The committee also

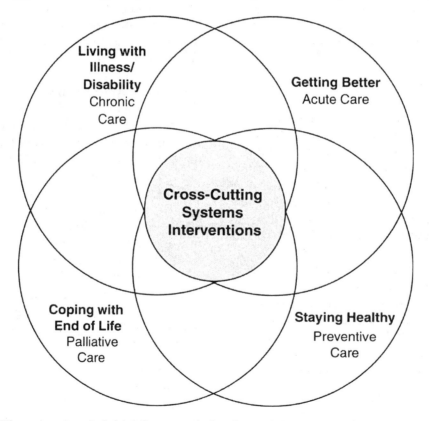

FIGURE 1-1 The committee's initial framework for determining priority areas.

---

[1] Terms in parentheses are the clinical terms corresponding to each of these stages.

recognized that a number of areas, such as the need for better coordination of care and support for self-management, cut across specific conditions and domains. The committee included these areas to emphasize the notion that changing the health system will require breaking down boundaries between diseases as well as classes of diseases. Thus, the committee supplemented the above four categories with a fifth—cross-cutting systems interventions—to ensure that improvement efforts will benefit all Americans, including those without specific priority conditions. Figure 1-1 presents the committee's initial framework. The overlapping circles represent the interrelatedness of the five categories.

Recommendation 1: The committee recommends that the priority areas collectively:

- **Represent the U.S. population's health care needs across the lifespan, in multiple health care settings involving many types of health care professionals.**

- **Extend across the full spectrum of health care, from keeping people well and maximizing overall health; to providing treatment to cure people of disease and health problems as often as possible; to assisting people who become chronically ill to live longer, more productive and comfortable lives; to providing dignified care at the end of life that is respectful of the values and preferences of individuals and their families.**

How Might the List of Priority Areas be Used?

The committee was acutely aware that report after report has been issued on the quality of health care and that government agencies and commissions have issued numerous "priority" recommendations. Another such report and list of priorities would not necessarily be helpful. The question is how this report is different and whether it might be a more practical guide to action.

Although it is impossible to predict all the activities that might be undertaken by various stakeholders to improve care in the priority areas identified by the committee, some uses of the list of areas presented in this report can be anticipated. These applications are likely to include the full range of health care system improvements and policy changes outlined in the *Quality Chasm* report, including applying evidence to health care, redesigning care processes around patient needs, making better use of information technology in the area of decision support, promoting accountability through measurement and performance feedback, and realigning payment incentives with quality care (Institute of Medicine, 2001a).

Building on the framework set forth in the *Quality Chasm* report, Berwick's (Berwick, 2002) *User's Guide for the IOM Quality Chasm Report* delineates four levels within the health care system at which quality improvement can take place (see Figure 1-2). Each priority area identified by the committee has aspects at each of these levels:

- Level A—the experience of patients

- Level B—the functioning of small units of care delivery, or micro-systems

- Level C—the functioning of organizations that support micro-systems

- Level D—the environment of policy, payment, regulation, accreditation, and other factors

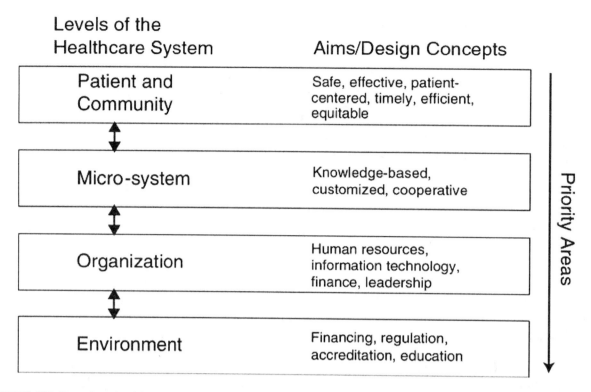

SOURCE: Reprinted with permission from Donald M. Berwick, M.D. (2002) (adapted from a slide used at the IOM Health Professions Education Summit held June 17-18, 2002 in Washington, D.C.).

FIGURE 1-2 Levels within the health care system for quality improvement.

Level A: The Experience of Patients

The overarching goal of quality improvement is to enhance the experience of patients. Achieving this goal entails improvement in the six national quality aims enumerated earlier: safety, effectiveness, patient-centeredness, timeliness, efficiency, and equity (Institute of Medicine, 2001a). While quality improvement generally involves reorganization at the levels of micro-systems, organizations, and environment, as described below, these efforts must ultimately be geared toward and judged by their ability to improve the direct experience of patients. Accordingly, one basis upon which the committee chose the priority areas was the degree to which broader changes in the way systems function in an area could improve the day-to-day care and quality of life for patients.

Level B: Micro-systems

Micro-systems are small work units that administer care to patients (Quinn, 1992). This "front-line" interaction is the basis on which patients judge their experience with the health care system. Examples of micro-systems include a physician' office, an intensive care unit, and an outpatient surgery center. This is the level that is closest to the direct needs of patients.

The Chronic Care Model provides one example of a multidimensional solution to the often chaotic structure found at the micro-system level (Improving Chronic Illness Care, 2002; Wagner, 2001; Wagner et al., 2001; Wagner et al., 1996). Developed at Group Health Cooperative of Puget Sound in the mid-1990s under the Improving Chronic Illness Care program of The Robert Wood Johnson Foundation, this model is focused on the care

Chronic Care Model

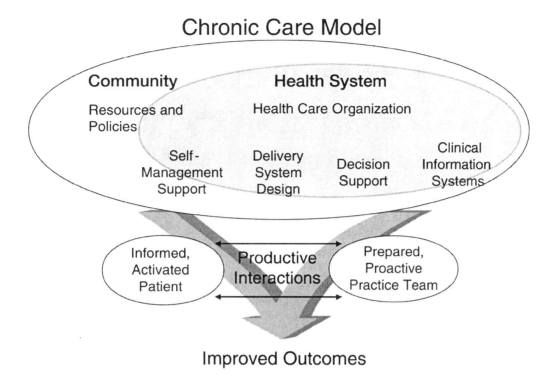

SOURCE: Reprinted with permission from Brian Austin (2002).

FIGURE 1-3 Chronic Care Model.

provided by primary care teams to patients with chronic illness and their families. Patients are expected to be active participants in their overall care plan and are acknowledged to be the principal managers of their condition(s). "Productive interactions" between an informed patient and a prepared practice team are the bedrock of the model. Patient preferences are emphasized, along with an evidence-based approach to effectively managing the course of the condition. Persistent planned follow-up completes the model. There are six key elements to this model, four of them implemented at the micro-system level (see Figure 1-3):

- Self-management support—recognition of the patient and family as the source of control, with the practice team collaborating and providing expertise and tools.

- Delivery system design—creation of a care

delivery structure appropriate to the planned management of patients with chronic illness, with clear roles for all staff.

- Decision support—integration of evidence-based guidelines into daily practice.

- Clinical information systems—reminder and feedback systems for clinicians and the tools to plan care for both individuals and whole populations of patients.

An example of the Chronic Care Model in action is the Health Disparities Collaboratives, spearheaded by the Bureau of Primary Health Care within DHHS (Health Disparities Collaboratives, 2002). The goal of these initiatives is to develop programs that expand access to high-quality, culturally and linguistically competent health care—both primary and preventive—for underserved, uninsured, and underinsured Americans, as well as those in traditionally underserved minority, ethnic, and racial groups. To meet this goal, the collaboratives focus on a subgroup of the entire population and then, if successful, spread to the rest of the patients in a community. The first collaborative, focused on diabetes, started in January 2000. Many of the priority conditions identified in this report could benefit from application of the Chronic Care Model. In addition to chronic care, the model's concepts could be applied in preventive (Glasgow et al., 2001), acute, and palliative care.

In the realm of pediatrics, a parallel model, referred to as the Medical Home, has been developed for children with special health care needs. In this model, the family, the physician, and other health professionals in the community constitute a team that is intimately involved in the management and facilitation of all aspects of pediatric care. The American Academy of Pediatrics defines the Medical Home as being accessible, continuous, comprehensive, family-centered, coordinated, compassionate, and culturally effective (The Medical Home, 2002). The basic principles behind the Chronic Care Model and the Medical Home offer unprecedented direction for transforming health care micro-systems.

Level C: Organizations

Care can also be improved at the level of the health care organization. Techniques for improving care within these broader systems include compiling a disease registry, facilitating access to evidence-based practice guidelines, ensuring that best practices are incorporated into daily procedures, and measuring outcomes and providing feedback on performance. The Veterans Administration's (VA) Quality Enhancement Research Initiative (QUERI) is an example of how a focus on priority areas can be used to change a health system by means of a data-driven, integrated quality improvement program. QUERI'S underlying goals are to identify best practices, to incorporate them into daily use, and to provide a feedback mechanism to ensure continuous quality improvement. The program functions to translate findings in the

research setting into improved patient care and system redesign (Demakis et al., 2000; Feussner et al., 2000; Kizer et al., 2000). A six-step process is employed to ensure systematic adherence to quality improvement efforts:

1. Identify high-risk/volume diseases among veterans.

2. Identify best practices.

3. Determine existing practice patterns and outcomes across VA and any current variation from best practices.

4. Identify and implement interventions to promote best practices.

5. Document the best practices that improve outcomes.

6. Document that outcomes are associated with improved health-related quality of life.

A first step in developing the program was to identify target conditions. Criteria used to determine this group of conditions included the number of veterans affected, the burden of illness, and known health risks within the veteran population. The conditions chosen for the initial efforts were chronic heart failure, diabetes, HIV/AIDS, ischemic heart disease, mental health (depression and schizophrenia), spinal cord injury, and stroke. The priority areas recommended in this report might similarly be used to guide organizational improvement efforts within other private and public health care organizations.

Level D: Environment

Health organizations operate within a broader financial and social environment that creates both incentives and constraints on how they operate. Even the best-intentioned and best-planned changes developed for patients and organizations will fail to be translated into real-world settings unless they are implemented in an environment containing the appropriate regulations and financial incentives. It is essential to consider these incentives when developing interventions to improve care in each of the priority areas. For example, payments might be bundled for management of some chronic conditions, or fee-for-service payments might be enhanced or tied to the achievement of certain performance goals for priority areas. Correspondingly, the priority areas identified in this report may represent particularly important focal points for the development and testing of models for better aligning these incentives with high-quality care.

Another important environmental influence is the educational system. Coordinating care and working cooperatively in interdisciplinary teams are not routinely emphasized in the training of health care professionals (Glick and Moore, 2001). As a result, clinicians often lack the necessary skills to effectively manage patients with chronic conditions. The priority areas can help drive the development of competency-based curricula that more closely mirror the demands of the practice environment.

What Can Be Expected from Those in the Field?

The committee readily acknowledges that there are organizations that have assumed leadership positions in many of the recommended priority areas. As part of its decision-making processes, the committee intentionally looked to the work of these groups. For example, as further discussed in chapter 4 and illustrated in Table 4-1, the committee selected seven chronic conditions that had already been targeted by other priority-setting initiatives.[2] The intent of the committee's list of priority areas is not to duplicate these efforts, but rather to promote synergy. The next step is to coordinate efforts and develop strategies for

these shared conditions. Such collective action will provide the necessary leverage for improvement in the priority areas to take hold. As noted earlier, to detect whether there has been a shift in the quality of the health care routinely received by Americans, AHRQ will monitor progress in these areas through the National Health Care Quality Report. The changes effected could be even more dramatic if groups already active in these areas, as well as those who have yet to become involved, were to join forces around the priority areas.

The selected priority areas also share common elements with other national efforts. For example, four of the leading health indicators[3] and ten of the focus areas[4] identified in Healthy People 2010 (HP2010) link directly to the priority areas (United States Department of Health and Human Services, 2000). Although this report supports the goals of HP2010—increasing quality and years of life and eliminating health disparities—the priority areas emphasize improving the health care delivery system, whereas HP2010 focuses on public health concerns.

The priority areas also coincide with many of the performance measures already in place to monitor health care quality. For example, the National Committee for Quality Assurance's (NCQA) Health Plan Employer Data and Information Set (HEDIS®), used to compare performance among managed care plans, contains measures relevant to 10 of the priority areas[5] (National Committee for Quality Assurance, 2002). The Joint Committee on Accreditation of Healthcare Organization's performance measurement initiative, ORYX, incorporates standardized performance measures into the accreditation process of

---

[2] Asthma, chronic obstructive pulmonary disease, diabetes, hypertension, ischemic heart disease, major depression, and stroke.

[3] Overweight and obesity, tobacco use, mental health, and immunizations.

[4] Cancer; diabetes; health communication; heart disease and stroke; immunization; maternal, infant, and child health; mental health; overweight; respiratory disease; and tobacco use.

[5] Antidepressant medication management, beta blocker treatment after heart attack, cervical cancer screening, childhood immunization status, cholesterol management after a heart attack, comprehensive diabetes care, controlling high blood pressure, follow-up after hospitalization for mental illness, prenatal and postpartum care, and use of appropriate medications for people with asthma.

hospitals. ORYX encompasses four core measurement areas on which hospitals must collect data for all patient discharges, all of which are applicable to the selected priority areas [6] (Joint Commission on Accreditation of Healthcare Organizations, 2002). As a final example, The Centers for Medicare and Medicaid Services (CMS) has implemented quality improvement organizations (QIOs) at the state and regional levels as a mechanism for improving the quality of care provided to Medicare beneficiaries (Centers for Medicare and Medicaid Services, 2002). The QIOs target six clinical topics, five of which overlap with the committee's priority areas.[7]

Even though there are many groups that implement performance measures, a common conceptual framework, such as the priority areas, is needed. At present there exists a patchwork of measures that often do not send consistent signals. Gains could be made in the standardization of these measures so that more meaningful and comparable quality-of-care information could be generated, thus reducing burden and contributing to greater improvements. The recently released IOM report *Leadership by Example: Coordinating Government Roles in Improving Health Care Quality* calls for the government to take the lead in promulgating standardized performance measures and points to the priority areas as the springboard for this effort (Institute of Medicine, 2002b).

In addition, it is the committee's hope that this report will be seen as a strong plea to physicians, nurses, pharmacists and other health care professionals, as well as health care organizations, to actively support and foster quality improvement in the priority areas identified herein. Each individual is encouraged to ask what he/she can do today, this month, this year to accelerate quality improvement in the priority areas in which he/she provides care.

First, everyone involved should recognize that the health care system will be changed only

through the individual and organized actions of patients, families, doctors, nurses, and administrators. All these groups must hold themselves accountable for making changes to improve the quality of the care they deliver or accept. And while it is recommended later in this report that AHRQ convene national experts to develop action plans for improvement in the priority areas, nobody involved should wait.

Second, the recommended priority areas deliberately encompass a wide range of health care issues in which improvement is necessary for overall system change. However, the priorities have been recommended, in part, so that most individuals and organizations can have a logical and much narrower focus. For example, patients and family members can focus on particular conditions that concern them. Patient-centered care requires engaged patients and families who understand the appropriate care recommendations and are willing and able to educate and challenge their providers if they are not receiving these services. Consumer and patient groups can and should focus on their particular conditions of interest, developing appropriate educational materials that support the most appropriate care; educating patients, providers, employers, policy makers, and the media about that care; and asking hard questions when it is not provided.

Likewise, providers, especially specialists, will usually regard one or more areas—whether it be diabetes or cancer screening or immunizations—as particular priorities. They can work to ensure that they are providing the best evidence-based care and that their colleagues are encouraged to do the same.

Health care organizations may deal with a broader array of issues, but again they can focus on certain priorities. For example, hospitals might start by addressing nosocomial infections, implementing the guidelines of the Centers for Disease Control and Prevention and ensuring through their associations and regulatory bodies that all hospitals implement those guidelines.

---

[6] Acute myocardial infarction, heart failure, community-acquired pneumonia, and pregnancy.
[7] Acute myocardial infarction, heart failure, stroke, diabetes management, pneumonia and influenza immunization.

Hospitals might also work to ensure that appropriate systems are in place to help doctors and nurses avoid pharmocolgical errors in the hospital and support clinicians in pain management.

Purchasers for both government and private programs should determine whether their coverage, payment, and information systems support and encourage health professionals in providing the clinically appropriate care at all times. Public- and private-sector policy makers should also work to identify data sources that clearly identify whether and where the appropriate care is and is not provided. The priority areas recommended by the committee may be a useful starting point for such efforts.

If quality improvement in the priority areas is to succeed, the collective efforts of all the aforementioned individuals and groups will need to be channeled into the effort. The *Quality Chasm* report recommends identification of the priority areas under the heading "Taking the First Steps" (Institute of Medicine, 2001a). The task is to take those first steps, and then continue the journey until we are confident that the quality chasm has been crossed.

Organization of the Report

Chapter 2 presents the rationale for the criteria used by the committee as a basis for selecting the priority areas. Chapter 3 identifies and describes the priority areas, including how they emerged from the selection process, the evidence base for their selection, and examples of how improving the quality of health care in these areas could have transformative impact on the quality of health care. Finally, Chapter 4 provides a detailed summary of the process developed and employed by the committee to identify candidate priority areas and narrow them down to the final list of 20 recommended in this report.

References

American Diabetes Association. "Facts & Figures: The Impact of Diabetes." Online. Available at http://www.diabetes.org/main/application/ commercewf;JSESSIONID_WLCS_DEFAULT http://www.diabetes.org/main/info/facts/impact/ default2.jsp [accessed Aug. 6, 2002].

Anderson, G., and J. R. Knickman. 2001. Changing the chronic care system to meet people's needs. *Health Aff (Millwood)* 20 (6):146-60.

Berwick, D. M. 2002. A User's Guide for the IOM's 'Quality Chasm' Report. *Health Aff (Millwood)* 21 (3):80-90.

Centers for Disease Control and Prevention. 2001. Trends in screening for colorectal cancer— United States, 1997 and 1999. *Morbidity and Mortality Weekly Report* 50:161-66.

———. 2002. *The Burden of Chronic Diseases and Their Risk Factors.* Atlanta, GA: CDC, National Center for Chronic Disease Prevention and Health Promotion.

Centers for Medicare and Medicaid Services. 2002. "Statement of Work, QIOs: 7th Round, February 2002 Version." Online. Available at http://www.hcfa.gov/qio/2b.pdf [accessed May 13, 2002].

Chassin, M. R. 1997. Assessing strategies for quality improvement. *Health Aff (Millwood)* 16 (3):151-61.

Chassin, M. R., and R. W. Galvin. 1998. The urgent need to improve health care quality. Institute of Medicine National Roundtable on Health Care Quality. *JAMA* 280 (11):1000-5.

Chassin, M. R., J. Kosecoff, R. E. Park, C. M. Winslow, K. L. Kahn, N. J. Merrick, J. Keesey, A. Fink, D. H. Solomon, and R. H. Brook. 1987. Does inappropriate use explain geographic variations in the use of health care services? A study of three procedures. *JAMA* 258 (18):2533-7.

Demakis, J. G., L. McQueen, K. W. Kizer, and J. R. Feussner. 2000. Quality Enhancement Research Initiative (QUERI): A collaboration between research and clinical practice. *Med Care* 38 (6 Suppl 1):I17-25 .

Feussner, J. R., K. W. Kizer, and J. G. Demakis. 2000. The Quality Enhancement Research Initiative (QUERI): From evidence to action. *Med Care* 38 (6 Suppl 1):I1-6.

Foundation for Accountability. 1997a. "The FACCT Consumer Information Framework: Comparative Information for Better Health Care Decisions." Online. Available at http://www.facct.org/information.html [accessed June 4, 2002a].

———. 1997b. *Reporting Quality Information to Consumers.* Portland, OR: FACCT.

Glasgow, R. E., C. T. Orleans, and E. H. Wagner. 2001. Does the Chronic Care Model serve also as a template for improving prevention? *Milbank Q* 79 (4):579-612, iv-v.

Glick, T. H., and G. T. Moore. 2001. Time to learn: The outlook for renewal of patient-centred education in the digital age. *Med Educ* 35 (5):505-9.

Harris Interactive. 2001. *Survey on Chronic Illness and Caregiving.* New York: Harris Interactive.

Health Disparities Collaboratives. 2002. "Health Disparities Collaboratives." Online. Available at http://www.healthdisparities.net/ [accessed June 4, 2002].

Hoffman, C., D. Rice, and H. Y. Sung. 1996. Persons with chronic conditions: Their prevalence and costs. *JAMA* 276 (18):1473-9.

Improving Chronic Illness Care. 2002. "Overview of the Chronic Care Model." Online. Available at http://www.improvingchroniccare.org/change/model/components.html [accessed June 4, 2002].

Institute of Medicine. 1999. *Ensuring Quality Cancer Care.* M Hewitt and J. V. Simone, eds. Washington, D.C.: National Academy Press.

———. 2000. *To Err Is Human: Building a Safer Health System.* L. T. Kohn, J. M. Corrigan, and M. S. Donaldson, eds. Washington, D.C: National Academy Press.

———. 2001a. *Crossing the Quality Chasm: A New Health System for the 21st Century.* Washington, D.C.: National Academy Press.

———. 2001b. *Envisioning the National Health Care Quality Report.* M. P. Hurtado, E. K. Swift, and J. M. Corrigan, eds. Washington, D. C.: National Academy Press.

———. 2002a. *Care Without Coverage: Too Little, Too Late.* Washington, D.C.: National Academy Press.

———. 2002b. *Leadership by Example: Coordinating Government Roles in Improving Health Care Quality.* Washington, D.C.: National Academy Press.

———. 2002c. *Unequal Treatment: Confronting Racial and Ethnic Disparities in Health Care.* B. S. Smedley, A. Y. Stith, and B. D. Nelson, Eds. Washington, D.C.: National Academy Press.

Joint Commission on Accreditation of Healthcare Organizations. 2002. "ORYX: The Next Evolution in Accreditation; Questions and Answers about the Joint Commission's Planned Integration of Performance Measures into the Accreditation Process." Online. Available at hhtp://www.jcaho.org/perfmeas/oryx_qa.html [accessed May 13, 2002].

Kizer, K. W., J. G. Demakis, and J. R. Feussner. 2000. Reinventing VA health care: Systematizing quality improvement and quality innovation. *Med Care* 38 (6 Suppl 1):I7-16.

Leatherman, S. and D. McCarthy. 2002. *Quality of Health Care in the United States: A Chartbook.* New York, NY: The Commonwealth Fund.

National Committee for Quality Assurance. 2002. *State of Health Care Quality Report.* Washington, DC: NCQA.

O'Connor, G. T., H. B. Quinton, N. D. Traven, L. D. Ramunno, T. A. Dodds, T. A. Marciniak, and J. E. Wennberg. 1999. Geographic variation in the treatment of acute myocardial infarction: The Cooperative Cardiovascular Project. *JAMA* 281 (7):627-33.

Partnership for Solutions, The Johns Hopkins University. 2001. "Partnership for Solutions: A National Program of The Robert Wood Johnson Foundation." Online. Available at http://www.partnershipforsolutions.org/statistics/prevalence.htm [accessed Dec. 12, 2002].

President's Advisory Commission on Consumer Protection and Quality in the Health Care Industry. 1998. *Quality First: Better Health Care for All Americans—Final Report to the President of the United States.* Washington DC: U.S. Government Printing Office.

Quinn, J. B. 1992. *Intelligent Enterprise: A Knowledge and Service Based Paradigm for Industry.* New York, N.Y.: New York Free Press.

Schuster, M. A., E. A. McGlynn, and R. H. Brook. 1998. How good is the quality of health care in the United States? *Milbank Q* 76 (4):517-63, 509.

The Medical Home. 2002. *Pediatrics* 110 (1 Pt 1):184-6.

United States Department of Health and Human Services. 2000. *Healthy People 2010.* In two volumes, conference edition. Washington, DC: U.S. Government Printing Office.

Wagner, E. H. 2001. Meeting the needs of chronically ill people. *BMJ* 323 (7319):945-6.

Wagner, E. H., B. T. Austin, C. Davis, M. Hindmarsh, J. Schaefer, and A. Bonomi. 2001. Improving chronic illness care: Translating evidence into action. *Health Aff (Millwood)* 20 (6):64-78.

Wagner, E. H., B. T. Austin, and M. Von Korff. 1996. Organizing care for patients with chronic illness. *Milbank Q* 74 (4):511-44.

Welch, W. P., M. E. Miller, H. G. Welch, E. S. Fisher, and J. E. Wennberg. 1993. Geographic variation in expenditures for physicians' services in the United States. *N Engl J Med* 328 (9):621-7.

Wennberg, J., and A. M. Gittelsohn. 1973. Small area variations in health care delivery. *Science* 182 (117):1102-8.

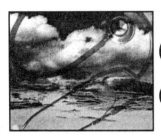

Chapter Two
Criteria for Selection

The committee's focus in determining selection criteria for the priority areas was on identifying a few core criteria that would lead to a list of areas representing opportunities to close gaps between known best practice and usual practice. Consistent with the *Quality Chasm* report, the committee started with the assumption that health care quality is a systems property that requires redesigning systems of care instead of just expecting health care workers to try harder (Institute of Medicine, 2001a). To date, most quality improvement efforts have been focused on changing the behavior of individual clinicians, often neglecting systems interventions (Mechanic, 2002). This report emphasizes such systems-level changes, although the committee also recognizes that improving quality requires work at multiple levels, including direct contact with clinicians and patients.

As noted in Chapter 1, the committee's immediate focus was on identifying the most promising opportunities for improving the delivery of existing best-practice treatments through changes in health care systems and policies, as distinct from efforts to improve the efficacy of existing best-practice treatments through continued biomedical research or technological innovation. Clearly, efforts to generate new scientific information for health care are critical. But unless we can develop more effective and efficient ways of delivering health care based on the best available known treatments, it is unlikely that such new knowledge will be used to its full benefit. As stated in the *Quality Chasm* report:

> At no time in the history of medicine has the growth in knowledge and technologies been so profound....[But] research on the quality of care reveals a health care system that frequently falls short in its ability to translate knowledge into practice, and to apply new technology safely and effectively.... If the health care system cannot consistently deliver today's science and technology, we may conclude that it is even less prepared to respond to the extraordinary scientific advances that will surely emerge in the first half of the 21st century (Institute of Medicine, 2001a:2-3).

Determining the criteria for the selection of priority areas required making choices and value judgments based on available evidence while taking into account principles of improving population health and effecting social justice. Several key questions had to be addressed. Should the emphasis be on conditions for which the potential for improvement through systems change is greatest, or those for which the clinical burden and quality deficits are greatest? What evidence is available to inform these decisions, and what are the gaps in that evidence? And what are the trade-offs between choosing priority areas for which the benefits are more modest but predictable and those for which the benefits are more uncertain but potentially greater?

The core issue underlying these questions—how best to allocate limited resources—is a question with which policy makers in the public and private sectors must grapple every day. The Institute of Medicine (IOM) has previously addressed priority setting in three other contexts—technology assessment (Institute of Medicine, 1992), clinical practice guidelines (Institute of Medicine, 1995), and research funding (Institute of Medicine, 1998a). However, this committee's charge was distinct from these previous efforts: to identify a set of conditions for which quality improvement within the health system could have the most benefit. Thus for candidate priority areas, the committee needed to examine:

- Not only the clinical burden of illness, but also the extent of preventable burden attributable to the failure to deliver best-practice care.

- Not just the degree to which the current system is broken, but also the extent to which known health care system changes could close gaps between best practice and usual care.

- Not only how to improve clinical care for the population as a whole, but also how to address unacceptable disparities in health care.

- Not only how to improve clinical care for individual conditions, but also how to identify an initial set of conditions for which improving care could be broadly transformative across the U.S. health care system.

General Considerations in Determining Criteria

The committee considered three general issues when discussing potential selection criteria. First, to what degree could existing evidence be a guide in assessing candidate priority areas according to the criteria? Second, how broadly should individual priority areas be defined? And finally, where should the line be drawn between the health care system and the rest of society in understanding the potential causes and consequences of the quality gaps in each area?

Determining Evidence and Measurability

It has been about 10 years since the term "evidence-based medicine" entered the medical literature (Guyatt, 1991), and since that time the term has become nearly ubiquitous in the vocabulary of clinicians, managers, and researchers. Evidence-based medicine involves the use of clinical research data to develop guidelines or best-practice standards for care. Just as evidence-based medicine can serve as a goal to guide clinical practice, the committee sought to ground its decisions, wherever possible, in quantitative data from the peer-reviewed literature and from nationally representative surveys.

While it is appealing to seek to apply the principles of evidence-based medicine to priority setting and quality improvement, a number of factors make doing so challenging for health systems (Walshe and Rundall, 2001). First, valid and widely applied measures do not exist for some exceptionally important concerns, such as functional capacity. As a result, available sources of data may not include essential gauges of the impact of some conditions in causing a loss of function or ability to cope with everyday situations, as opposed to the resulting mortality. Although there are cross-sectional and longitudinal data on functional status available at the national[1] and state levels[2] these surveys provide only population-specific information and are not linked to particular interventions. Second, there is a considerably smaller evidence base for the impact of systems-based quality improvement efforts than for more traditional efforts to improve treatment efficacy for particular clinical conditions, as the former type of work is very difficult to accomplish. Third, even if more data were available, many of the most important decisions—such as how to weigh the potential for far-reaching improvements against the needs of the sickest individuals—cannot be made using quantitative data. Rather, addressing such matters requires a qualitative approach that explicitly emphasizes principles of social justice and equity.

Thus, the committee sought to incorporate the broadest possible range of evidence into its decision-making process, but to have at each step of the process a clear understanding of the sources and potential limitations of that evidence. Similarly, while it was essential for the selection of priority areas to be based on strong evidence of the existence of quality problems, it was also critical to find scientific evidence that a particular intervention in an area can result in improvement and that accurate, valid, and reliable measures to document that improvement are available and can be collected at a reasonable cost. Thus, some conditions that have a major impact on morbidity or mortality were excluded from the initial set of candidate areas because there is no strong evidence of effective interventions for them, or there are no adequate measures to indicate when improvement has occurred. Where potentially important data were lacking, this report provides recommendations for conducting further research.

Balancing Breadth and Focus

The committee sought to balance breadth and focus in defining particular priority areas. If the areas were defined broadly enough (e.g., infectious disease, chronic illnesses), it would literally have been possible to construct a list of 15 to 20 areas that included almost every condition. However, using such broad categories would likely have resulted in quality improvement efforts that were diffuse and ultimately ineffective. On the other hand, focusing on narrowly defined conditions might mean squandering an opportunity to effect more systemic change or failing to address areas across the entire age spectrum. In considering the appropriate level of specificity for the priority areas, the committee sought to identify areas that, give the available evidence, could serve as a basis for achieving meaningful quality improvement over the next 3 to 5 years.

Defining the Boundaries of the Health System

A final issue that inevitably arises in setting health care priorities is where to draw the line between the health system and the rest of society. Thus while it is known that poverty is one of the strongest and most persistent predictors of ill health, it is less clear whether or to what degree addressing this concern falls within the purview of health policy (Deaton, 2002; Marmot, 2002). In dealing with this issue, the committee considered the burden of illness and potential benefits of quality improvement from the broadest possible perspective, including benefits accruing not only to patients, but also to families, employers, and society as a whole. In keeping with the committee's charter, however, the health system, rather than other forms of societal intervention, was considered the primary potential engine for such improvement. In addressing the problem of tobacco use, for example, tobacco counseling by health

---

[1] National Health Interview Survey (Centers for Disease Control and Prevention, 2002b); MEPS (Medical Expenditure Panel Survey, 2002); Medicare Expenditure Survey (Centers for Medicare and Medicaid Services, 2002).
[2] Behavioral Risk Factor Surveillance System (Centers for Disease Control and Prevention, 2002a).

providers, not cigarette taxes or antismoking campaigns, would be the focus for health care system–based quality improvement (Rigotti, 2002). On the other hand, the potential benefits of such counseling were considered from a broad societal perspective.

In this connection, the committee did not explicitly examine strategies for improving access to health care or eliminating disparities in care. Two other IOM reports—*Care Without Coverage: Too Little, Too Late* (Institute of Medicine, 2002a) and *Unequal Treatment: Confronting Racial and Ethnic Disparities in Health Care* (Institute of Medicine, 2002b)— focus explicitly on these problems. However, the committee did examine unwarranted variation in the delivery of quality care based on socioeconomic status, race/ethnicity, age, gender, and other demographic factors. For example, issues of the stigma associated with mental health care and of health literacy were addressed.

Criteria for Selecting the Priority Areas

The committee identified and used three interdependent criteria—impact, inclusiveness and improvability—for selecting the priority areas. Applied together, these criteria were intended to result in a set of priority areas for which quality improvement could be transformative to the U.S. health care system, resulting in wide-ranging, sustainable changes in other areas.

Impact comprises the extent of the burden—including disability, premature death, and economic costs—imposed by a condition with respect to quality and quantity of life for patients, as well as for families, employers, and society as a whole.

Improvability focuses on the degree to which gaps and unwarranted variations in the delivery of evidence-based medical care could be eliminated through changes in an area, and on opportunities to achieve major improvements in the heath care system by addressing the six national aims of quality improvement defined in the *Quality Chasm* report as being most important to patients and their families: safety, effectiveness, patient-centeredness, timeliness, efficiency, and equity (Institute of Medicine, 2001a). Core aspects of improvability include: (1) the existence of evidence-based standards or guidelines for effective care, (2) the availability of reliable measures that can be applied to understand and close gaps in care, (3) documented (measured, known) and unwarranted variations in care, and (4) examples of circumstances in which system changes have been applied successfully to close gaps in care.

Inclusiveness involves the applicability of the priority areas to a broad range of patients across the life span from birth to death, with particular emphasis on redressing disparities and social inequities in care and not leaving vulnerable groups behind. In addition, this criterion is defined to ensure that the full spectrum of health care services (from preventive to palliative care) would be included in an area and that a variety of health care settings, organizations, and providers would be engaged in any national health care quality improvement effort in that area.

Table 2-1 summarizes the criteria chosen by the committee for selecting priority areas for health care improvement. Each criterion is discussed in detail in the following subsections.

Recommendation 2: The committee recommends use of the following criteria for identifying priority areas:

- *Impact*—**the extent of the burden— disability, mortality, and economic costs—imposed by a condition, including effects on patients, families, communities, and societies.**

TABLE 2-1 Criteria for Selecting the Priority Areas for Quality Improvement

Criteria	Defining Questions	Chief Considerations
Impact	How big is the problem?	**Patient and family impact:** Clinical burden of illness and quality gaps; psychosocial effect on patients and caregivers; consumer dissatisfaction with care quality **System impact:** Health care system burden; health care provider burden; costs **Societal impact:** Burden on society outside of the health care system
Improvability	Are there significant gaps between best practice and usual care and unwarranted variations in care? Is there evidence that existing quality gaps and variations in care can be narrowed or eliminated?	**Condition improvability:** Best-practice treatment or standard; valid and reliable measures for understanding and eliminating variations **System improvability:** Opportunity to improve relative to six aims of the Quality Chasm report; efficacy and cost-effectiveness of efforts to close quality gaps; existing and emerging areas **Health disparity improvability:** Opportunity to narrow gaps in care and disease burden for vulnerable and disadvantaged populations
Inclusiveness	Will addressing the priority area improve quality of care for a broad spectrum of patients and health care settings? Will the priority area result in improved health and quality of life for persons who are otherwise at a disadvantage in health care?	**Patient inclusiveness (breadth, reach, and equity):** Age, gender, race/ethnicity, socioeconomic status, geographic location **Condition inclusiveness:** Preventive care, acute care, chronic care, palliative care **Health care system inclusiveness:** Intervention directed at multiple settings and constituents: inpatient and outpatient, providers, managers/policy makers

- *Improvability*—the extent of the gap between current practice and evidence-based best practice and the likelihood that the gap can be closed and conditions improved through change in an area; and the opportunity to achieve dramatic improvements in the six national quality aims identified in the *Quality Chasm* report (safety, effectiveness, patient-centeredness, timeliness, efficiency and equity).

- *Inclusiveness*—the relevance of an area to a broad range of individuals with regard to age, gender, socioeconomic status, and ethnicity/race (equity); the generalizability of associated quality improvement strategies to many types of conditions and illnesses across the spectrum of health care (representativeness); and the breadth of change effected through such strategies across a range of health care settings and providers (reach).

Impact: How Big Is the Problem?

The criterion of impact seeks to quantify the magnitude of the burden imposed by a particular condition at both the individual and population levels. Clinically, the burden imposed can be quantified in terms of prevalence (how many people have the condition), premature mortality (how many years of life are lost because of the condition and because of shortcomings in its treatment), and morbidity (the extent to which the condition affects function and quality of life). Summary measures—such as disability-adjusted life years (DALYs), which combines years of life lost as a result of premature death with years lived with disability (World Health Organization, 2000), and quality-adjusted life years—have been developed to combine length and quality of life into a single metric (Coffield et al., 2001; Fryback, 1998; Maciosek et al., 2001). For the health system, burden can be estimated using cost and quality data.

Impact has been the criterion used most frequently in previous priority-setting efforts. Earlier IOM reports have identified prevalence, burden of illness, and cost as key criteria for technology assessment and guideline development (Institute of Medicine, 1992; Institute of Medicine, 1995). The Medical Expenditure Panel Survey uses prevalence and cost in identifying its list of priority conditions (Cohen, 2001). Similarly, prevalence, mortality, disability, quality of life, and cost are central criteria used by the National Institutes of Health for assessing the distribution of research funding (Gross et al., 1999; Institute of Medicine, 1998a).

Why Look at Impact?

Two arguments can be made for the importance of impact as a complement to improvability in setting priorities. First, gaps in evidence on improvability can potentially be filled by data on disease impact. That is, in the absence of clear evidence on effectiveness, it can reasonably be assumed that conditions imposing the greatest burden potentially represent the greatest need for improvement. Similarly, since a small portion of the population incurs the vast majority of health expenditures in the United States (Berk and Monheit, 2001), targeting improvement toward high-cost populations/conditions could yield widespread change in the health system.

Second, even if one can show that a condition is improvable, a measure of impact is necessary to ensure a level of equity in the distribution of the resources devoted to improvement. Strict adherence to cost-effectiveness, or the "greatest good for the greatest number," can lead to a crowding out of life-saving treatments by interventions that provide small benefit to a large portion of the population. For instance, during one priority-setting process, an initial approach focusing on cost-effectiveness analysis resulted in tooth capping being assigned a higher priority than appendectomy (Hadorn, 1991).

In contrast to this utilitarian calculus, egalitarian approaches seek to balance such considerations with attention to the least well off (Brock, 2002; Olsen, 1997). For receipt of clinical care, the least well off can be defined in at least two ways—patients who are the sickest and those who may be at particularly high risk of receiving poor-quality care. Similarly, data on cost and quality can be used to determine those potential priority areas for which the system is most in need of improvement.

To balance the above approaches, the committee examined impact using three broad types of evidence—estimates for clinical health and disease burden, estimates for system health and gaps in quality, and evidence on disparities in care.

Measuring Impact with Reference to Population Health

In 1998 an IOM panel addressed the critical issue of how best to measure health and illness across populations (Institute of Medicine, 1998b). The panel concluded that population health measures clearly need to account for both mortality and morbidity, but that more work was needed to understand how best to combine the two into summary measures. The panel suggested that while some of the limitations of existing summary measures were methodological, others represented the fact that "all measures of population health involve choices and value judgments in both their construction and application" (Institute of Medicine, 1998b:12). Therefore, the panel encouraged "side-by-side" comparisons of different measures, informed by an understanding of the assumptions involved in each (Institute of Medicine, 1998b:20).

In keeping with those previous recommendations, the committee examined a number of sources of data for understanding the impact of disease on population health. For each candidate priority area, the committee examined data on mortality from the National Center for Health Statistics (Minino and Smith, 2001) and on prevalence and disability from the Medical Expenditure Panel Survey (Medical Expenditure Panel Survey, 1997). The committee also considered current estimates for DALYs. Rather than seeking to combine these data for a single ranking, the committee examined the assumptions underlying each measure and the similarities and differences among them. The committee also recognized some of the shortcomings of the data sources used, including inherent biases in determining the quality of a person's life and the focus of most datasets on diseases as opposed to health status and functionality. These datasets focus on diseases because the clinical literature is organized around diseases as well as the health care system—hence the prevalence of specialists. Thus, it difficult to create an evidence framework that starts from symptoms or functioning.

How "Broken" is the Health System?

In addition to focusing on the clinical burden of disease, the committee looked at the degree to which the health system is "broken" with regard to how it cares for a particular condition. The committee used two measures—cost-of-illness data and national quality

information—to identify those conditions for which system problems are the most pronounced. The committee reviewed cost data from the Medical Expenditure Panel Survey, examining costs for both specific conditions and groupings of particular relevance (e.g., patterns of costs for multiple chronic conditions). For each potential priority area, the committee looked at total population expenditures, average expenditures among affected individuals, and the gap between total expenditures and disability.

To examine quality of care across the range of candidate areas and begin to identify those areas with the greatest potential improvability, the committee examined data from the National Committee for Quality Assurance's (NCQA) State of Managed Care Report, which rates health plans that collectively cover 90 percent of Americans enrolled in health maintenance organizations (HMOs) (National Committee for Quality Assurance, 2001). Areas in which variation across plans was largest and in which care most consistently fell short of performance goals were identified as potential candidates for quality improvement.

Improvability: Can the Problem Be Fixed?

Improvability reflects the degree to which existing gaps in the use of proven best practices can be closed for a priority area through system and policy changes that can lead to better care and better outcomes, including improved health, productivity, and quality of life. Improvability also encompasses the opportunity to achieve dramatic improvements in the six quality aims identified in the *Quality Chasm* report, enumerated above (Institute of Medicine, 2001a).

Evidence for Improvability

Improvability originates in the premise that an effective (and potentially cost-effective) treatment has been identified, but that this treatment is not delivered in safe or appropriate ways to all those who need it. Applying this criterion requires evidence not only for an effective best-practice treatment, but also for the potential to eliminate existing quality gaps or unwarranted variations in clinical practice in ways that could be widely replicated throughout the health care system in both public and private settings and among a broad range of patient and provider populations.

Under ideal circumstances, evidence for improvability would include supporting data for both the efficacy and cost-effectiveness of feasible system and policy improvements. However, existing studies of health care quality improvement initiatives provide very little data on the relative efficacy or cost-effectiveness of various types of system and policy change. The committee considered the existence of valid and reliable measures for assessing the processes and outcomes of care to be a major asset in efforts to guide and monitor health care system improvement.

Cost-Effectiveness Analysis in Priority Setting

Cost-effectiveness analysis has typically been the starting point for economic models of priority setting (Weinstein et al., 1996) and was the method used in the first version of the Oregon Medicaid process. Such analysis seeks to determine how, given limited financial resources, health resources should be allocated to maximize health benefits.

While appealing from a conceptual perspective, the committee identified substantial limitations in relying excessively on cost-effectiveness estimates for its priority-setting process. First, a review of the current literature comparing cost-effectiveness across interventions (Harvard School of Public Health, 2002) showed that few studies meet criteria designed to ensure interpretability and comparability among estimates (Rigotti, 2002; Siegel et al., 1996). Second, the gaps in the literature are particularly notable for chronic conditions such as diabetes, chronic obstructive pulmonary disease, and asthma, all of which were potential priority areas for the committee.

Third, even for conditions for which such analyses are available, treatments range widely in cost-effectiveness, making it difficult to summarize overall improvability for care within particular priority areas. Fourth, there are a number of special populations for whom information is scarce, such as children, the medically indigent, and those receiving home-based care. Finally, the vast majority of cost-effectiveness studies have focused on clinical treatments rather than quality improvement or system change. For this report, as noted earlier, quality improvement is defined not as a function of the development of new treatment methods or technologies, but as of the deployment of existing methods and technologies more widely and effectively through health system redesign (Chassin and Galvin, 1998).

The Agency for Healthcare Research and Quality and private organizations such as The Robert Wood Johnson Foundation are currently leading efforts to foster more rigorous studies of the effectiveness of quality improvement initiatives. As yet, however, few such studies exist (Renders et al., 2001; Schoenbaum et al., 2001; Wells et al., 2000). Generalizing findings and comparing results across interventions will likely be a complex undertaking, given how sensitive the interventions are to the context of the systems in which they are implemented. However, it will be essential to attempt to synthesize the data as they become available. For example, the U.S. Preventive Services Task Force recently published its findings from a systematic review of the literature examining the cost-effectiveness of colorectal screening. Although screening for colorectal cancer was found to be cost-effective (between $10,000 and 25,000 per life-year saved) the question of what screening method or methods are best remains unanswered (Pignone et al., 2002; United States Preventive Services Task Force, 2002).

Thus, while the committee did examine cost and cost-effectiveness data, it had to rely more on studies examining the efficacy and effectiveness of clinical treatments than on data regarding the cost-effectiveness of alternative system-based quality improvement strategies.

Because most studies typically use disease-specific outcome measures, they were more useful for ensuring that effective treatments are available than for ranking improvability across candidate priority areas. For understanding potential improvability, then, the committee supplemented quantitative research with case studies of successful efforts to improve systems of care within each of the candidate priority areas.

Inclusiveness: Breadth, Reach, and Equity

It is essential not only to examine the impact and improvability of candidate priority areas, but also to address the issue of inclusiveness: the mix of areas, the populations affected, and opportunities to address inequities in health care and health status in the United States. This criterion reflects the committee's strong belief that the priority list needs to include areas relevant to children and adults, rich and poor, and urban and rural populations. It is also important to focus on conditions for which there are particularly large disparities in care between the general population and vulnerable racial, ethnic, economic, or geographic populations. Given the goal of broad health system change, the committee also believed it important to select priority areas that would involve interventions across different sectors and specialties within the health care delivery system. In addition, the committee wanted to ensure that the list of areas would be representative across the four broad domains of health care enumerated in Chapter 1—preventive, acute, chronic, and palliative (Institute of Medicine, 2001b). Indeed, inclusiveness considerations helped motivate the decision to include some cross-cutting areas among the priority areas to ensure that national quality improvement efforts would in some way benefit all Americans and all health care systems and providers.

Transformative Potential

The end product of the above three criteria is a set of priority areas with the potential to transform the health care system. The concept of transformative potential reflects the extent to which the priority areas, both individually and collectively, are likely to catalyze far-reaching and sustainable changes by perturbing the current system in a way that helps trigger a self-corrective course. More specifically, the concept has to do with the extent to which improvements in the delivery of care in one priority area could extend beyond this initial target to generate changes in other areas. Such influence could occur because one condition (e.g., diabetes) may be a risk factor for multiple other conditions (e.g., blindness, renal failure, artherosclerosis), or because system changes, such as creating a patient reminder system, if implemented in one area, could also improve care for other conditions. Similarly, system changes required, for instance, to integrate tobacco dependence treatment into routine care could stimulate similar improvements in other preventive services. With regard to palliative care, system changes designed to engender and document advanced care plans could be used for every fatal illness. In addition, improvements in some areas might serve as leverage points or requirements in other areas. For example, improvements in health literacy are needed to promote active patient self-management for most conditions.

REFERENCES

Berk, M. L., and A. C. Monheit. 2001. The concentration of health care expenditures, revisited. *Health Aff (Millwood)* 20 (2):9-18.

Brock, D. 2002. Priority to the worst off in health care resource prioritizations. *Chapter 28 in Medicine and Social Justice.* R. Rhodes, M. P. Battin, and A. Silvers, eds. New York, NY: Oxford University Press.

Centers for Disease Control and Prevention. 2002a. "Behavioral Risk Factor Surveillance System." Online. Available at http://www.cdc.gov/brfss [accessed Oct. 15, 2002a].

————. 2002b. "National Health Interview Survey (NHIS)." Online. Available at http://www.cdc.gov/nchs/nhis.htm [accessed Oct. 15, 2002b].

Centers for Medicare and Medicaid Services. 2002. "The Medicaire Current Beneficiary Survey (MCBS)." Online. Available at http://cms.hhs.gove/mcbs/default.asp [accessed Oct. 15, 2002].

Chassin, M. R., and R. W. Galvin. 1998. The urgent need to improve health care quality. Institute of Medicine National Roundtable on Health Care Quality. *JAMA* 280 (11):1000-5.

Coffield, A. B., M. V. Maciosek, J. M. McGinnis, J. R. Harris, M. B. Caldwell, S. M. Teutsch, D. Atkins, J. H. Richland, and A. Haddix. 2001. Priorities among recommended clinical preventive services. *Am J Prev Med* 21 (1):1-9.

Cohen, S. B. 2001. Enhancements to the Medical Expenditure Panel Survey to improve health care expenditure and quality measurement. In Proceedings of the Statistics in Epidemiology Section, American Statistical Association.

Deaton, A. 2002. Policy implications of the gradient of health and wealth. An economist asks, would redistributing income improve population health? *Health Aff (Millwood)* 21 (2):13-30.

Fryback, D. G. 1998. Methodological issues in measuring health status and health-related quality of life for population health measures: A brief overview of the "DALY" family of measures. In *Summarizing Population Health: Directions for the Development and Application of Population Metrics.* M. J. Field and M. R. Gold, eds. Washington, D.C.: National Academy Press.

Gross, C. P., G. F. Anderson, and N. R. Powe. 1999. The relation between funding by the National Institutes of Health and the burden of disease. *N Engl J Med* 340 (24):1881-7.

Guyatt, G. H. 1991. Evidence-based medicine. *ACP J Club* 114:A-16.

Hadorn, D. C. 1991. Setting health care priorities in Oregon: Cost-effectiveness meets the rule of rescue. *JAMA* 265 (17):2218-25.

Harvard School of Public Health. 2002. "The CUA Data Base: Standardizing the Methods and Practices of Cost-Effectiveness Analysis." Online. Available at http://www.hsph.harvard.edu/organizations/hcra/cuadatabase/intro.html [accessed May 29, 2002].

Institute of Medicine. 1992. *Setting Priorities for Health Technologies Assessment: A Model Process.* M. S. Donaldson and H. C. Sox, Jr., eds. Washington, D.C.: National Academy Press.

————. 1995. *Setting Priorities for Clinical Practice Guidelines.* M. J. Field, eds. Washington, D.C.: National Academy Press.

————. 1998a. *Scientific Opportunities and Public Needs: Improving Priority Setting and Public Input at the National Institutes of Health.* Washington, D.C.: National Academy Press.

————. 1998b. *Summarizing Population Health: Directions for the Development and Application of Population Metrics.* M. J. Field and M. R. Gold, eds. Washington, D.C.: National Academy Press.

————. 2001a. *Crossing the Quality Chasm: A New Health System for the 21st Century.* Washington, D.C.: National Academy Press.

————. 2001b. *Envisioning the National Health Care Quality Report.* M. P. Hurtado, E. K. Swift, and J. M. Corrigan, eds. Washington, D.C.: National Academy Press.

————. 2002a. *Care Without Coverage: Too Little, Too Late.* Washington, D.C.: National Academy Press.

————. 2002b. *Unequal Treatment: Confronting Racial and Ethnic Disparities in Health Care.* B. S. Smedley, A. Y. Stith, and B. D. Nelson, Eds. Washington, D.C.: National Academy Press.

Maciosek, M. V., A. B. Coffield, J. M. McGinnis, J. R. Harris, M. B. Caldwell, S. M. Teutsch, D. Atkins, J. H. Richland, and A. Haddix. 2001. Methods for priority setting among clinical preventive services. *Am J Prev Med* 21 (1):10-9.

Marmot, M. 2002. The influence of income on health: Views of an epidemiologist. Does money really matter? Or is it a marker for something else? *Health Aff (Millwood)* 21 (2):31-46.

Mechanic, D. 2002. Improving the quality of health care in the United States of America: The need for a multi-level approach. *J Health Serv Res Policy* 7 (3 Suppl):35-9.

Medical Expenditure Panel Survey. 1997. *Panel Population Characteristics and Utilization Data for 1996.* AHCPR Publication 98-DP12. Rockville, MD: Agency for Health Care Policy and Research.

————. 2002. "Introduction to MEPS Data and Publications." Online. Available at http://www.meps.ahcpr.gov/Data_Public.htm [accessed June 4, 2002].

Minino, A. M. and B. L. Smith. 2001. *National Vital Statistics Reports.* Centers for Disease Control and Prevention.

National Committee for Quality Assurance. 2001. *The State of Managed Care Quality.* Washington, D.C.: NCQA.

Olsen, J. A. 1997. Theories of justice and their implications for priority setting in health care. *J Health Econ* 16 (6):625-39.

Pignone, M., S. Saha, T. Hoerger, and J. Mandelblatt. 2002. Cost-effectiveness analyses of colorectal cancer screening: A systematic review for the U.S. Preventive Services Task Force. *Ann Intern Med* 137 (2):96-104.

Renders, C. M., G. D. Valk, S. J. Griffin, E. H. Wagner, J. T. Eijk Van, and W. J. Assendelft. 2001. Interventions to improve the management of diabetes in primary care, outpatient, and community settings: A systematic review. *Diabetes Care* 24 (10):1821-33.

Rigotti, N. A. 2002. Clinical practice: Treatment of tobacco use and dependence. *N Engl J Med* 346 (7):506-12.

Schoenbaum, M., J. Unutzer, C. Sherbourne, N. Duan, L. V. Rubenstein, J. Miranda, L. S. Meredith, M. F. Carney, and K. Wells. 2001. Cost-effectiveness of practice-initiated quality improvement for depression: Results of a randomized controlled trial. *JAMA* 286 (11):1325-30.

Siegel, J. E., M. C. Weinstein, L. B. Russell, and M. R. Gold. 1996. Recommendations for reporting cost-effectiveness analyses. Panel on Cost-Effectiveness in Health and Medicine. *JAMA* 276 (16):1339-41.

United States Preventive Services Task Force. 2002. "Recommendations and Rationale: Screening for Colorectal Cancer." Online. Available at http://www.ahrq.gov/clinic/3rduspstf/colorectal/colorr.htm [accessed Nov. 20, 2002].

Walshe, K., and T. G. Rundall. 2001. Evidence-based management: From theory to practice in health care. *Milbank Q* 79 (3):429-57, IV-V.

Weinstein, M. C., J. E. Siegel, M. R. Gold, M. S. Kamlet, and L. B. Russell. 1996. Recommendations of the Panel on Cost-effectiveness in Health and Medicine. *JAMA* 276 (15):1253-8.

Wells, K. B., C. Sherbourne, M. Schoenbaum, N. Duan, L. Meredith, J. Unutzer, J. Miranda, M. F. Carney, and L. V. Rubenstein. 2000. Impact of disseminating quality improvement programs for depression in managed primary care: A randomized controlled trial. *JAMA* 283 (2):212-20.

World Health Organization. 2000. "Global Burden of Disease 2000 Version 1 Estimates." Online. Available at http://www3.who.int/whosis/menu [accessed May 29, 2002].

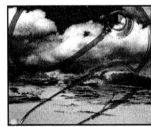 # Chapter 3
Priority Areas for
Quality Improvement

The committee's deliberations led to the selection of 20 priority areas for health care quality improvement:

- Care coordination (cross-cutting)

- Self-management/health literacy (cross-cutting)

- Asthma—appropriate treatment for persons with mild/moderate persistent asthma

- Cancer screening that is evidence-based—focus on colorectal and cervical cancer.

- Children with special health care needs[1]

- Diabetes—focus on appropriate management of early disease

- End of life with advanced organ system failure—focus on congestive heart failure and chronic obstructive pulmonary disease

- Frailty associated with old age—preventing falls and pressure ulcers, maximizing function, and developing advanced care plans

- Hypertension—focus on appropriate management of early disease

- Immunization—children and adults

- Ischemic heart disease—prevention, reduction of recurring events, and optimization of functional capacity

[1] The Maternal and Child Health Bureau defines this population as "those (children) who have or are at increased risk for a chronic physical, developmental, behavioral or emotional condition and who also require health and related services of a type or amount beyond that required by children generally" (McPherson et al., 1998:138).

- Major depression—screening and treatment

- Medication management—preventing medication errors and overuse of antibiotics

- Nosocomial infections—prevention and surveillance

- Pain control in advanced cancer

- Pregnancy and childbirth—appropriate prenatal and intrapartum care

- Severe and persistent mental illness—focus on treatment in the public sector

- Stroke—early intervention and rehabilitation

- Tobacco dependence treatment in adults

- Obesity (emerging area)[2]

The committee made no attempt to rank order the priority areas selected. The first 2 listed above—care coordination and self-management/health literacy—are cross-cutting areas in which improvements would benefit a broad array of patients. The 17 that follow represent the continuum of care across the life span and are relevant to preventive care, inpatient/surgical care, chronic conditions, end-of-life care, and behavioral health, as well as to care for children and adolescents. Finally, obesity is included as an "emerging area" that does not at this point satisfy the selection criteria as fully as the other 19 priority areas.

This chapter first reviews the breadth of opportunities for health care improvement represented by the committee's recommended list of priority areas. The three types of areas included on the list—cross-cutting areas, specific conditions, and emerging areas—are then described. The chapter next profiles each area in detail, including the aim of intervention in that area and the rationale for the area's selection in light of the three criteria discussed in Chapter 2—impact, improvability and inclusiveness.

Breadth of Opportunities Represented by Priority Areas

The priority areas selected by the committee can be viewed through a variety of lenses. They represent a range of health care services and challenges, including:

- The full spectrum of health care, from preventive and acute care, to chronic disease management, to long-term and palliative care at the end of life. Thus they encompass a wide variety of health care services, spanning both reactive acute, emergency, and surgical care and the proactive planned care required to prevent and manage chronic disease, pain, and disability.

- Care provided for a variety of populations representing Americans of all ages and demographic groups, including care that is oriented to individuals and families, as well as populations.

- Care delivered in a range of publicly and privately financed ambulatory and inpatient health care settings (outpatient and community health centers, home-based care, emergency departments, hospitals, and nursing homes) by a variety of health care practitioners (physicians, nurses, pharmacists, allied health professionals), including both generalists and specialists.

The Full Spectrum of Health Care

As noted, the priority areas recommended by the committee represent health care quality improvement challenges and opportunities across the full spectrum of health care. In fact, having relevance to multiple domains of care strengthened an area's chances of being included on the final list. Boxes 3-1 to 3-6 show how the priority areas relate to a wide range of health care needs. For example, ischemic heart disease figures prominently in preventive care, inpatient/surgical care, chronic

---

[2] An emerging area is one of high burden (impact) that affects a broad range of individuals (inclusiveness) and for which the evidence base for effective interventions (improvability) is still forming.

care, and end-of-life care. Similarly, medication management cuts across inpatient/surgical care, chronic care, end-of-life care, and child/adolescent care. Obesity—the emerging area—touches on preventive care, chronic care, behavioral health, and child/adolescent care.

The Entire Life Span

The committee made a concerted effort to ensure that the priority areas selected would represent issues pertinent to all age groups. Figure 3-1 shows how the priority areas cut across the stages of a typical life span. As demonstrated, only a few areas are unique to certain age groups, such as children with special health care needs and frailty prevention and management. Many areas, such as cancer screening and hypertension, cluster around adulthood and extend into end of life. Additionally, nine of the priority areas encompass the entire life span.

Diverse Health Care Settings and Professions

The set of priority areas recommended by the committee involves care that is provided in multiple health care settings and organizations, care that is both privately and publicly funded, and care that is provided by a variety of health care professionals. For example, effective asthma management requires integration of care among primary care providers, pediatricians, schools, hospitals (particularly emergency rooms), and pharmacists. Adequate pain control in advanced cancer and stroke rehabilitation require a continuum of care that includes home, community, clinic, and hospital. Improving quality of care for severe and persistent mental illness, such as psychosis, provides an opportunity to focus on the effectiveness of mental health services provided by the public sector (Narrow et al., 2000; Wells, 2002a). To close the gaps between best practice and usual care for the full set of proposed areas will require the collective expertise of a vast array of doctors, nurses, pharmacists, allied health professionals, social workers, and vested laypersons. Virtually every conventional medical specialty will need to develop strategies for one or more of these priority areas.

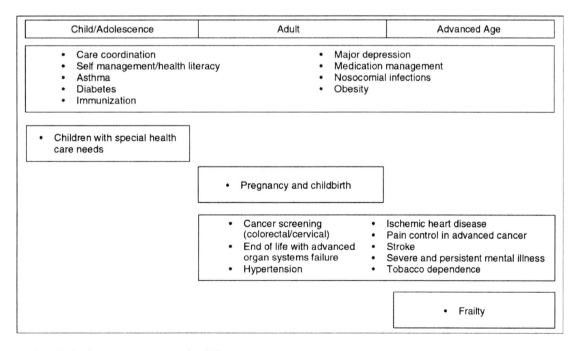

Figure 3-1: Priority areas across the life span.

Box 3-1 Priority Areas That Relate to Preventive Care

- Care coordination (cross-cutting)
- Self-management/health literacy (cross-cutting)
- Cancer screening
- Hypertension
- Immunization
- Ischemic heart disease (prevention)
- Major depression (screening)
- Pregnancy and childbirth
- Tobacco dependence
- Obesity (emerging area)

Box 3-2 Priority Areas That Relate to Behavioral Health

- Care coordination (cross-cutting)
- Self-management/health literacy (cross-cutting)
- Major depression
- Severe and persistent mental illness
- Tobacco dependence
- Obesity (emerging area)

Box 3-3 Priority Areas That Relate to Chronic Conditions

- Care coordination (cross-cutting)
- Self-management/health literacy (cross-cutting)
- Asthma
- Children with special health care needs
- Diabetes
- End of life with advanced organ system failure
- Frailty
- Hypertension
- Ischemic heart disease

- Major depression (treatment)
- Medication management
  - Medication errors
  - Overuse of antibiotics
- Pain control in advanced cancer
- Severe and persistent mental illness
- Stroke
- Tobacco dependence
- Obesity (emerging area)

Box 3-4 Priority Areas That Relate to End of Life

- Care coordination (cross-cutting)
- Self-management/health literacy (cross-cutting)
- Chronic conditions
- End of life with advanced organ system failure
- Frailty
- Medication management
  - Medication errors
  - Overuse of antibiotics
- Nosocomial infections
- Pain control in advanced cancer

Box 3-5 Priority Areas That Relate to Children and Adolescents

- Care coordination (cross-cutting)
- Self-management/health literacy (cross-cutting)
- Asthma
- Children with special health care needs
- Diabetes
- Immunization (children)
- Major depression
- Medication management
  - Medication errors
  - Overuse of antibiotics
- Obesity (emerging area)

Box 3-6 Priority Areas That Relate to Inpatient/Surgical Care

- Care coordination (cross-cutting)
- Self-management/health literacy (cross-cutting)
- End of life with advanced organ system failure
- Ischemic heart disease
- Medication management
  - Medication errors
  - Overuse of antibiotics
- Nosocomial infections
- Pain control in advanced cancer
- Pregnancy and childbirth
- Severe and persistent mental illness
- Stroke

Three Types of Priority Areas

Cross-Cutting Areas

There was strong consensus among the committee members on the critical need to improve care coordination, support for self-management, and health literacy for all patients and their families. System and policy changes to achieve improvement in these cross-cutting priority areas would involve most health care organizations and practitioners, could impact all types of conditions, and could provide a means of dramatically improving health care for all Americans.

Improved care coordination would, if applied broadly, have an especially important impact on improving health care processes and outcomes for children and adults with serious chronic illness and multiple chronic conditions (Anderson and Knickman, 2001; Anderson, 2002b). Efforts to improve health literacy are in turn essential for effective self-management and collaborative care. For example, a recent study found that diabetics with poor health literacy, unable to read and/or comprehend directions on their pill bottles, had worse blood sugar control and higher rates of preventable vision impairment (Schillinger et al., 2002). Devising strategies to improve health literacy—both at the micro level, where patients and health care professionals interact, and at the macro level, where population health is the target—would not only improve diabetes outcomes, but also form part of a package of improvements for nearly all inadequate aspects of health care.

Specific Priority Conditions

Chronic Care

In keeping with the *Quality Chasm* report, which notes the critical need to close quality gaps for the growing numbers of Americans with chronic disease (Institute of Medicine, 2001a), the majority of the specific priority conditions recommended are chronic. For all of the recommended conditions, such as diabetes, hypertension, and ischemic heart disease, there are known, effective interventions that can be applied to improve health outcomes, reduce disease burden, and prevent more serious health problems later in life. Moreover, the enormous and rapid growth in the prevalence and burden of chronic disease over the past two decades has been a major force in clarifying the limitations of the current health care system—which evolved primarily to meet acute and emergency health care needs—thus motivating broad action for health care system redesign (Bodenheimer et al., 2002; Institute of Medicine, 2001a).

Acute Care

One priority area within the realm of acute care—effective medication management—focuses on preventing medication errors and the overprescribing of antibiotics, particularly for acute respiratory infections in children. This area provides an excellent opportunity for designing interventions that can enhance the use and capacity of management information systems. For example, lecturing to physicians about medical errors yields small gains, but technological advances, such as the electronic medical record tied to computerized medication orders with acceptable dosage ranges and interactions, can dramatically reduce errors arising from incorrect orders (Bates et al., 1999; Kaushal et al., 2001). Computerized alerts of potential drug interactions, prompts and reminders for required services, and electronic physician order entry for prescriptions could all be put in place to safeguard health and improve quality of care (Hunt et al., 1998). Corrective measures that redesign work so that errors are "engineered out" are repeatedly found to have high leverage.

Preventive Care

The committee explicitly included preventive services among the domains of health care that should be represented by the priority areas. Doing so reflected a growing body of evidence that early detection and timely intervention for risk factors or diseases in their preclinical stages are effective in reducing both disease burden and costs. Selected priority areas represent a range of clinical preventive services involving immunization, screening, and counseling for lifestyle changes, which would singly and collectively reduce morbidity and mortality due to the nation's leading chronic illnesses and infectious disease threats. Specifically, childhood/adult immunization, improved screening for colorectal and cervical cancers, and brief primary care interventions for adult tobacco dependence have been identified as major opportunities for cost-effective improvements in the nation's health care system (Coffield et al., 2001).

For example, just 3–5 minutes of counseling and medication advice given to adult smokers by their physician could more than double the quitting success rates smokers achieve on their own (Fiore et al., 2000). Since there are over 430,000 tobacco-related deaths each year from heart disease, stroke, lung cancer, and chronic lung disease among U.S. adults, the impact of this simple intervention, combined with other effective modes of tobacco treatment, would be dramatic (Max, 2001; United States Department of Health and Human Services, 2000). Unfortunately, only about 50 percent of patients who smoke receive such advice and assistance, largely because supports such as office-based reminder systems and insurance coverage for smoking cessation services are not widely in place (Goodwin et al., 2001; Thorndike et al., 1998). Treating tobacco dependence is critical to preventing disease in healthy populations of smokers, the progression of illnesses caused by tobacco use, poor pregnancy outcomes associated with smoking, and pediatric asthma in infants and adolescents whose parents smoke. Furthermore, there is growing evidence that the types of system and policy changes needed to spur broader use of evidence-based tobacco interventions are similar to those required to support the wider delivery of other proven interventions for changes in health behavior in primary care, such as counseling on physical activity and diet and on the importance of reducing risky consumption of alcohol

(Glasgow et al., 2001).

Palliative Care

Between 2010 and 2030, America's baby boomers will move beyond the age of 65 and swell the number of older persons to approximately 70 million, representing 20 percent of the population (Administration on Aging, 2002). Accordingly, the committee placed particular emphasis on addressing the complex care issues that surface after age 65 and particularly after age 80. One of the priority areas in the category of palliative care is frailty. Nearly everyone who survives past age 80 experiences a period of frailty involving decreased functional status as a result of multiple health problems, such as heart and lung disease, as well as cognitive deficits resulting from dementia or stroke. As more and more Americans face the physical and social challenges of frailty, systems of care must adapt in ways that allow them to live comfortably and safely at home. Advanced care plans should be put in place that are respectful of both the patient's and family's wishes. This priority area can serve as an exemplar for health care quality improvements that incorporate changes at various levels of the health care delivery system to provide integrated, dignified care for those of advanced age.

Emerging Areas

Obesity was intentionally placed last on the committee's list and classified as an "emerging area." The prevalence of overweight and obesity among Americans has reached epidemic proportions (Mokdad et al., 2001; Yanovski and Yanovski, 2002). Obesity represents an important medical condition in its own right and contributes to morbidity and mortality for other diseases, including heart disease, type II diabetes, osteoarthritis, hypertension, and cancer. Addressing growing rates of obesity and obesity-related disease in children and adults has been identified as an urgent national health care priority (Squires, 2001).

Obesity was selected as a priority area based on strong evidence for its impact and inclusiveness, but still emerging evidence for improvability. That is, there was relatively limited evidence for the efficacy of existing best-practice treatments for obesity in children and adults, such as behavioral counseling and drug and surgical interventions (Epstein et al., 2001). In addition, effective treatment for obesity will need to integrate many other aspects of society, such as housing, exercise opportunities, food supply, and work patterns, often considered outside the traditional realm of health care.

The committee's aim in denoting obesity as "emerging" was to accelerate the rate at which research generates the evidence needed to identify effective interventions and to develop evidence-based treatment guidelines and valid performance measures. Since this area would serve as a model for potential future emerging priority areas, formal reviews of progress on obesity would be conducted more frequently than for other priority areas, perhaps as often as yearly, to determine future directions.

Priority Areas: Detailed Descriptions

The following brief descriptions are intended as illustrative rather than exhaustive profiles for each of the 20 recommended priority areas. The committee's goal was to provide a starting point for experts in the field to undertake effective national health care quality improvement efforts over the next 3 to 5 years. Each priority area is discussed with reference to the committee's three selection criteria—impact, improvability, and inclusiveness. A vignette is also provided for selected areas to illustrate how a transformed health care system would provide quality care in that area.

Care Coordination

Aim

To establish and support a continuous healing relationship, enabled by an integrated clinical environment and characterized by the proactive delivery of evidence-based care and follow-up. Clinical integration is further defined as "the extent to which patient care services are coordinated across people, functions, activities, and sites over time so as to maximize the value of services delivered to patients" (Shortell et al., 2000:129).

Rationale for Selection

Impact

Nearly half of the population—125 million Americans—lives with some type of chronic condition. About 60 million live with multiple such conditions. And more than 3 million—2.5 million women and 750,000 men—live with

five such conditions (Partnership for Solutions, 2001). For those afflicted by one or more chronic conditions, coordination of care over time and across multiple health care providers and settings is crucial. Yet in a survey of over 1,200 physicians conducted in 2001, two-thirds of respondents reported that their training was not adequate to coordinate care or education for patients with chronic conditions (Partnership for Solutions, 2001).

More than 50 percent of patients with hypertension (Joint National Committee on Prevention, 1997), diabetes (Clark et al., 2000), tobacco addition (Perez-Stable and Fuentes-Afflick, 1998), hyperlipidemia (McBride et al., 1998), congestive heart failure (Ni et al., 1998), chronic atrial fibrillation (Samsa et al., 2000), asthma (Legorreta et al., 2000), and depression (Young et al., 2001) are currently managed inadequately. Among the Medicare-eligible population, the average beneficiary sees 6.4 different physicians in a year, 4.6 of those being in the outpatient setting (Anderson, 2002a).

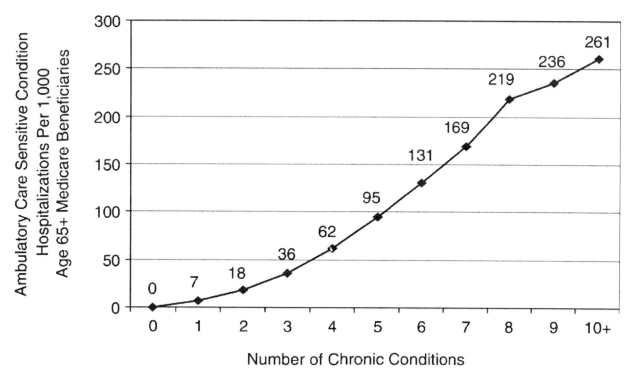

SOURCE: Reprinted with permission from Gerard Anderson, Ph.D. (2002).

Figure 3-2. Hospitalizations among Medicare beneficiaries with multiple chronic conditions.

Among this same population, as the number of chronic conditions a person has increases, so, too, does the number of hospitalizations that are inappropriate or avoidable because outpatient treatment would have been effective: from 7 per 1,000 for those with one chronic condition to 95 per 1,000 for those with five chronic conditions and 261 per 1,000 for those with ten or more such conditions (Anderson, 2002a). See Figure 3-2.

Improvability

In a randomized controlled trial of 970 patients with diabetes cared for by over 450 primary care providers, usual care was compared with a program utilizing regular follow-up, decision support, reminder systems, and modern self-management support. After 6 years, patients in the intervention group had significantly better outcomes, including lower HbA1c, blood pressure, and cholesterol levels (Olivarius et al., 2001). A recent review of ambulatory-care diabetic management programs found that patient education and an expanded role for a nurse in the intervention strategy also improved patient outcomes (Renders et al., 2001).

According to a meta-analysis of adult immunization and cancer screening programs, interventions that had the largest impact involved organizational changes, such as the use of a planned care visit for prevention, and designation of nonphysician staff to carry out specific prevention activities (Stone et al., 2002). There is also a growing body of evidence that planned (e.g., proactive, structured) care at set intervals makes a difference, and can be accomplished using nonstandard models, such as group visits (Beck et al., 1997; Sadur et al., 1999).

The Chronic Care Model, described in Chapter 1, provides a structure for planned, clinically integrated care. There are promising indications that a wide variety of health systems can reorganize themselves to deliver such care (The National Coalition on Health Care and the Institute for Healthcare Improvement, 2002; Wagner et al., 2001a).

Inclusiveness

The Institute of Medicine's 2002 report *Unequal Treatment: Confronting Racial and Ethnic Disparities in Health Care* documents racial and ethnic disparities in several of the priority areas recommended in this report, all of which could benefit from a more integrated approach to care. These areas include children with special health care needs, diabetes, end of life with advanced organ system failure, frailty, pregnancy and childbirth, and severe and persistent mental illness (Institute of Medicine, 2002).

Box 3-7 Care Coordination

One participating organization, Care Management Group of Greater NY, Inc. (CMGNY), in the Institute for Healthcare Improvement and The Robert Wood Johnson Foundation's National Program on Improving Chronic Illness Care incorporated the elements of the Chronic Care Model to enhance recognition and treatment of depression in patients with congestive heart failure. This collaborative is an excellent example of how effective care coordination, or clinical integration of services, improved health outcomes for the chronically ill, particularly for patients with multiple chronic conditions.

First, there was strong organizational support from key leaders at CMGNY, a subsidiary of the North Shore Long Island Jewish Health System. Second, clinical information systems were used to extract claims data and a disease registry was built to identify patients within the plan who had been diagnosed with congestive heart failure (CHF). Physicians participating in the program were given the names of their CHF patients for systematic screening for depression. Patients with recent hospitalizations, patients identified through care management, and patients whose annual costs exceeded $50,000 per year, were all targeted for depression assessment as well. Third, decision support was provided at many levels. Physicians within the plan were invited to attend "managed care college" where they were trained to recognize the classic signs of depression and coached to administer the Patient Health Questionnaire (PAQ), a screening tool for depression. Notably, clinicians were given financial incentives for incorporating the PAQ into their daily practice. Additionally, primary care physicians had access to a psychiatrist by telephone for consultation regarding medication dosage and depression management. Fourth, a nurse practitioner used telephone self-management support techniques to facilitate partnerships between patients and their providers. The hallmark of this relationship was active listening and empathy with the overarching goal to educate the patient about their condition and to monitor and encourage adherence to their treatment plan, including medications and appointments. In addition, goal-setting strategies were developed with the patient to encourage exercise and engagement in pleasant events as well as to resolve treatment-emergent problems such as side effects from antidepressant medications, attitudinal issues and social barriers. Fifth, the overall delivery of care was redesigned to incorporate elements of the chronic illness care model, including care management, decision support and development of community relationships. This included providing services outside the doctor's office such as home health evaluations, home psychiatric evaluations, physical therapy and a home health aide. A nurse practitioner figured prominently in coordinating, monitoring and following-up of care. Lastly, patients were linked with community resources both on the local and national level.

Outcomes from this study were dramatic. After 6 months a 50 percent or greater improvement in depression severity was observed among participants. In the words of one patient with CHF who was clinically depressed and on 20 medications "you have turned my life around" (Cole et al., 2002; Cole, 2002).

Self-Management/Health Literacy

Aim

To ensure that the sharing of knowledge between clinicians and patients and their families is maximized, that the patient is recognized as the source of control, and that the tools and system supports that make self-management tenable are available.

Self-management support is defined as the systematic provision of education and supportive interventions to increase patients' skills and confidence in managing their health problems, including regular assessment of progress and problems, goal setting, and problem-solving support. Health literacy is defined as the ability to read, understand, and act on health care information. Specifically, improvement in this area encompasses four features of successful programs: (1) providers communicate and reinforce patients' active and central role in managing their illness; (2) practice teams make regular use of standardized patient assessments; (3) evidence-based programs are used to provide ongoing support; and (4) collaborative care planning and patient-centered problem solving result in an individualized care plan for each patient and support from the team when problems are encountered (Glasgow et al., 2002).

Rationale for Selection

Impact

According to the National Adult Literacy Survey, 40–44 million of the 191 million adults (21 percent) in the United States are functionally illiterate: they read at or below the fifth-grade level or cannot read at all (American Medical Association, 2002). Another 50 million adults (25 percent of adult Americans) are marginally literate: they are able to locate and assimilate information in a simple text, but are unable to perform tasks that require them to assimilate or synthesize information from complex or lengthy texts (American Medical Association, 2002). The *Journal of the*

American Medical Association reported in 1999 that 46 percent of American adults are functionally illiterate in dealing with the health care system (American Medical Association, 2002). Patients with low literacy are frequently ashamed and hide it. A 1996 study of patients with reading difficulty confirmed that 67 percent had never told their spouse and 19 percent had never told anyone about their reading problem (American Medical Association, 2002).

People with low literacy skills have to rely on remembering what health professionals tell them. Recall of medical instructions is often poor; one study showed that people remembered only 14 percent of spoken instructions for managing fever or sore throat (Pfizer, 1998). A 1997 study of patients in two public hospitals found that those with inadequate literacy skills were five times more likely to misinterpret their prescriptions than patients with adequate reading skills, and averaged two more doctor visits per year than those with marginal or adequate literacy skills (American Medical Association, 2002). In one study, 23 percent of English-speaking and 34 percent of Spanish-speaking respondents were found to have an inadequate ability to read and comprehend medical information in their spoken language. Furthermore, of those with low ability to read medical information, only 55 percent reported having someone in their household who could read for them (Pfizer, 1998).

The estimated additional health care expenditures due to low health literacy skills total about $73 billion. Employers may be financing as much as 17 percent of these additional expenditures (American Medical Association, 2002).

Improvability

Self-management support is critical because patients and their families are the primary caregivers in chronic illness (Von Korff et al., 1997). There is evidence that in the current system, even minimal health education is inadequate for people with chronic illness: just 45 percent of persons with diabetes received formal education on managing their condition in 1998; 42 percent of patients with a diagnosis of cardiovascular disease, diabetes, or hyperlipidemia received counseling or education on diet and nutrition in 1997; and 8.4 percent of patients with asthma received formal patient education in 1998 (United States Department of Health and Human Services, 2000). However, more than education is required for outcome change to occur. As noted by Norris (Norris et al., 2001) in a systematic review of diabetes self-management training: "It is apparent that factors other than knowledge are needed to achieve long-term behavioral change. . . and improved personal attitudes and motivations are more effective than knowledge in improving metabolic control in type II diabetes."

There is strong evidence that support for self-management is a critical success factor for chronic disease programs. For example, a meta-analysis of primary care diabetes programs found that 19 of 20 interventions including a self-management component had improved a process or outcome of care (Renders et al., 2001). In addition, a study that investigated the effect of self-management education and regular practitioner review for adults with asthma demonstrated a statistically significant reduction in the proportion of subjects reporting hospitalizations and emergency room visits , unscheduled doctor visits, days lost from work, and episodes of nocturnal asthma (Gibson et al., 2000). A companion review analyzed trials that employed only limited education interventions and concluded that education did not have a significant effect unless it was coupled with an action plan, self-monitoring or regular review (Gibson et al., 2002).

With regard to health literacy, use of both written and verbal communication has been shown to be the most effective way of increasing patient understanding and compliance. (American Medical Association, 2002). Research with junior college students, for example, showed that recall of spoken medical instructions was enhanced by having pictographs representing those instructions

present during learning and recall (Pfizer, 1998). The fact that the Hispanic subjects in the study did especially well in recalling pictograph meanings suggests that this approach may be helpful with groups for whom English is a second language.

Several measures of literacy have been found to correlate significantly with comprehension. The time spent reading sample leaflets and finding answers to questions about the documents was positively and significantly associated with comprehension measured by a true–false test. Two pronunciation measures and a literacy test based on correctly defining drug terminology also correlated significantly with true–false test comprehension (American Medical Association, 2002).

Inclusiveness

Poor health literacy is a widespread problem that affects people of all social classes and from all ethnic groups. Functional health literacy is worst among the elderly and low-income populations, impacting more than 66 percent of U.S. adults aged 60 and over and approximately 45 percent of all adults who live in poverty. Thus, the populations most in need of health care are least able to read and understand information needed to function as a patient (American Medical Association, 2002; United States Department of Health and Human Services, 2000).

Appropriate Treatment for Persons with Mild/Moderate Persistent Asthma

Aim

To ensure that all persons with mild/moderate persistent asthma receive appropriate treatment with pharmacotherapy and suitable self-management support.

Rationale for Selection

Impact

It is estimated that in the United States, 14.6 million persons have active asthma (Centers for Disease Control and Prevention, 2001a). In 1999, an estimated 478,000 persons were hospitalized (Centers for Disease Control and Prevention, 1999b) and 2 million sought emergency care for acute asthma exacerbations (Centers for Disease Control and Prevention, 1999a). While death from asthma is almost always considered preventable, over 4,600 persons in the United States died from this condition in 1999 (United States Department of Health and Human Services, 2002).

In 1998, the economic burden associated with asthma was estimated at $12.7 billion annually. This figure includes nearly $7.4 billion in direct health care expenditures and an additional $5.3 billion in indirect costs. Loss of school days alone accounts for nearly $1.1 billion annually (Weiss and Sullivan, 2001). The inflation-adjusted costs of asthma have risen over the past decade (Weiss et al., 2000). Despite these increases in costs, however, there have been few clear signs that health care for those with asthma has substantively improved.

Numerous studies published throughout the 1990s and as recently as 2001 reveal that guidelines for asthma care are not being followed (Diette et al., 2001; Hartert et al., 2000; Legorreta et al., 1998). A number of national public and private agencies continue to recognize the suboptimal care and clinical outcomes for this disease. The United States Department of Health and Human Services

(DHHS), through its Healthy People 2010 initiative, calls for reductions in asthma hospitalization rates (United States Department of Health and Human Services, 2000). The National Committee for Quality Assurance (NCQA) has added a performance measure to the Health Plan Employer Data and Information Set (HEDIS) that is aimed at improving the use of anti-inflammatory medications for persons with persistent asthma (National Committee for Quality Assurance, 1997). Most recently, the American Medical Association has focused on the importance of improving of asthma care through its physician-based measures (Antman, 2002).

The use of antiinflammatory medications and asthma education, including the provision of self-management support, are essential to improved asthma care. However, a number of studies suggest that health system redesign may also be required to optimally improve asthma care and thereby clinical outcomes (Evans et al., 1999; Greineder et al., 1999; Mayo et al., 1990; Zeiger et al., 1991). Studies such as the recently reported work of the Pediatric Asthma Care Patient Outcomes Research Team suggest that provider education alone will not significantly improve asthma outcomes without system redesign through a planned asthma care approach (Finkelstein et al., 2002).

Improvability

Since the late 1980s, there has been mounting evidence of substantial variations in asthma care and of the inadequate or suboptimal nature of much of the care provided (Diette et al., 2001; Hartert et al., 2000; Legorreta et al., 1998). In response to this problem, in 1987 the National Asthma Education and Prevention Program of the National Heart, Lung, and Blood Institute convened a national expert panel to develop guidelines for the treatment of the disease. These guidelines, first published in 1991 (National Asthma Education and Prevention Program, 1991) and updated in 1997 (NHLBI USPHS, 1997) and 2002 (NAEPP Expert Panel Report, 2002), provide a benchmark by which to view the current practice of asthma care.

One of the cornerstones of these guidelines is the use of anti-inflammatory medications for the treatment of persons with persistent asthma. A number of different medications make up this therapeutic group, and of these, inhaled corticosteroids have been recommended as the preferred therapy (NHLBI USPHS, 1997). There are also a number of other key elements to the guidelines, few of which are as commonly agreed upon as the need to provide asthma education focused on support for self-management of the disease (NHLBI USPHS, 1997).

Inclusiveness

Afflicting more than 14 million persons, asthma is a disease that affects all segments of the population—children and adults, males and females, urban and rural populations, and the wealthy and the poor (Centers for Disease Control and Prevention, 2001a). At the same time, perhaps the most important problem related to asthma care is the disproportionate impact of poor care on minority populations and persons of lower socioeconomic status (Centers for Disease Control and Prevention, 1998; Grant et al., 2000).

Asthma meets the inclusiveness criterion as it relates to the health care system. Care for persons with asthma extends across the primary care specialties of pediatrics, family medicine, and internal medicine. It also is an important health care concern for two subspecialty groups—allergists and pulmonolgists. Within asthma care, there are important lessons for outpatient, emergency department, and hospital-based care.

Cancer Screening That Is Evidence-Based

Aim

To enhance the effectiveness of screening programs designed to prevent colorectal and cervical cancer. More specifically, the aims are to increase the number of individuals who are offered appropriate screening for these cancers and to ensure that timely follow-up is provided.

In this report, colorectal and cervical cancer are used as examples, with the goal that effective systems-based interventions implemented for these two cancers could serve as models for other cancers where an evidence base is documented for screening or could be used once one has been established.

Rationale for Selection

Impact

Colorectal cancer is the third most common cancer among men and women in the United States, with an estimated incidence of 148,300 cases annually. In 2002, 56,600 Americans died from colorectal cancer, making it the nation's second leading cause of cancer-related death. Lifetime risk for developing colorectal cancer is approximately 6 percent with over 90 percent of cases occurring after age 50 (American Cancer Society, 2002). The estimated long-term cost of treating stage II colon cancer is approximately $60,000 (Brown et al., 2002).

Cervical cancer is the ninth most common cancer among women in the United States, with an estimated incidence of 13,000 cases annually. Cervical cancer ranks thirteenth among all causes of cancer death, with about 4,100 women dying of the disease each year (American Cancer Society, 2002). The incidence of cervical cancer has steadily declined, dropping 46 percent between 1975 and 1999 from a rate of 14.8 per 100,000 women to 8.0 per 100,000 women (Ries et al., 2002). Despite these gains, cervical cancer continues to be a significant public health issue. It has been estimated that 60 percent of cases of cervical cancer are due to a lack of or deficiencies in screening (Sawaya and Grimes, 1999).

Improvability

Early diagnosis of colorectal cancer while it is still at a localized stage results in a 90 percent survival rate at 5 years (Ries et al., 2002). The American Cancer Society's (ACS) guidelines recommend screening for colorectal cancer beginning at age 50 for adults at average risk using one of the following five screening regimens: fecal occult blood test (FOBT) annually; flexible sigmoidoscopy every 5 years; annual FOBT plus flexible sigmoidoscopy every 5 years; double contrast barium enema every 5 years; or colonoscopy every 10 years (American Cancer Society, 2001). The United States Preventive Services Task Force strongly recommends screening for men and women 50 years of age and or older for colorectal cancer. Screening has been found to be cost-effective in saving lives, with estimates ranging from $10,000 and $25,000 life-year saved. However, data were insufficient to determine whether one screening strategy is superior to another (Pignone et al., 2002; United States Preventive Services Task Force, 2002b).

In a nationally conducted survey assessing current rates of use of colorectal screening tests, 40.3 percent of respondents reported having had FOBT and 43.8 percent sigmoidoscopy or colonscopy at some point in time. With regard to screening being done within recommended ACS guidelines, 20.6 percent of respondents reported having FOBT within 1 year, and 33.6 percent reported having had sigmoidoscopy or colonoscopy within 5 years (Seeff et al., 2002). Another national survey found that between 1992–1998 only a slight increase was observed in screening for colorectal cancer, and in 1998, only 22.9 percent of respondents age 50 or older had been screened with a home administered FOBT in the past year or proctoscopy within 5 years (Nadel et al., 2002).

Widespread use of the Papanicolaou (Pap) test over the past 50 years as a screening tool for cervical cancer has led to an estimated 70 percent decline in mortality from this disease

(Dewar et al., 1992; Saslow et al., 2002). Early detection of cervical cancer that is still localized results in a 5-year survival rate of 92 percent (American Cancer Society, 2002). The American Cancer Society's guidelines recommend that cervical cancer screening should start 3 years after a woman begins having sexual intercourse, but not later than 21 years of age, given that cervical cancer risk has been associated with sexually transmitted infection with certain types of human papilloma virus (HPV). Subsequently, women should have a Pap test every 3 years (American Cancer Society, 2002; Saslow et al., 2002). A recently report controlled trial demonstrated that administration of a HPV vaccine reduced both the incidence of HPV infection as well as HPV related cervical cancer among study participants (Koutsky et al., 2002).

As of 2000, the median percentage of women who had had a Pap test within the past 3 years was 86.8 percent (Centers for Disease Control and Prevention, 2000a). Despite these high screening rates, more than 50 percent of women in the United States who develop cervical cancer have either never undergone screening or not done so within the 3 years prior to diagnosis (NIH Consensus Statement, 1996). These women are likely to be older, to live in rural communities, and to be of low socioeconomic status (Anderson and May, 1995). Immigrant women with limited English proficiency are at especially high risk of never undergoing screening (Harlan et al., 1991).

Outcomes of a 5-year demonstration project targeting low-income members of minority groups who received their health care through the Los Angles County Department of Health Services demonstrated that systems-level strategies increased cervical cancer screening rates among this traditionally high-risk group. Systems interventions included physician education to heighten awareness of screening guidelines; patient education regarding risk factors for cervical cancer; policy interventions, such as written protocols to ensure follow-up of abnormal results; and expanded capacity, for example, increased clinic hours and same-day

appointments for referrals. During the intervention time period, patients were three times more likely to receive screening as compared with the base line year (Bastani et al., 2002).

Ambiguity among health plans regarding coverage for cancer screening is a systems-related barrier. A study in which insurance departments were queried nationally found that 28 states and Puerto Rico did not require coverage for cervical cancer screening. Lack of consensus pertaining to guideline use was also demonstrated. Fourteen states and the District of Columbia have adopted ACS guidelines for cervical cancer screening whereas seven states have elected to use nonconforming guidelines (Rathore et al., 2000).

Inclusiveness

African Americans have the highest incidence of and mortality from colorectal cancer among racial/ethnic groups. Their mortality rate from the disease is 22.8 per 100,000 in the U.S. population and is at least double that of Asians/Pacific Islanders (10.7 per 100,000), American Indians/Alaskan Natives (10.3 per 100,000), and Hispanics (10.2 per 100,000) (American Cancer Society, 2002).

Vietnamese women have the highest age-adjusted incidence rate for cervical cancer (43 per 100,000) as compared with Japanese women, who have the lowest rate (15 per 100,000). Three ethnic groups have incidence rates of 15 per 100,000 or higher—Alaska Natives, Koreans, and Hispanics. African American women have an incidence rate of 13.2 per 100,000 for cervical cancer as compared with Caucasian women with a rate of 8.7 per 100,000. Mortality rates are also higher among African Americans than Caucasians, at 6.7 per 100,000 and 2.5 per 100,000, respectively (National Cancer Institute, 1996). African Americans are less likely than Caucasians to have their cervical cancer diagnosed at an early stage, with 44 percent of invasive cancers being diagnosed at a localized stage for the former as compared with 56 percent for the latter (American Cancer Society, 2002).

Children with Special Health Care Needs

Aim

To maximize the quality of care for children with special health care needs by addressing key processes of care, including care planning; use of preventive services; access to specialists, ancillary services, mental health services, and dental services; and care coordination.

The Maternal and Child Health Bureau defines this population as "those (children) who have or are at increased risk for a chronic physical, developmental, behavioral or emotional condition and who also require health and related services of a type or amount beyond that required by children generally" (McPherson et al., 1998:138).

Rationale for Selection

Impact

Although children with special health care needs having substantial medical problems make up a relatively small proportion of the pediatric population, it is particularly important to focus on (1) maximizing the quality of their health care, because they are the most in need of services, and (2) increasing the cost-effectiveness of their health care, because it is the most expensive. In recent years, the prevalence of complex chronic conditions has dramatically increased even as medical, surgical, and technological advances have decreased the mortality rates for infants, children, and adolescents (Cadman et al., 1987; Gortmaker et al., 1990; Ireys, 1981; Newacheck et al., 1991; Newacheck et al., 1998; Newacheck and Taylor, 1992). Among the total pediatric population, it is estimated that 6.7 percent have significant activity limitations, 0.2 percent have a limitation in an essential activity, such as eating, bathing, or dressing; and 0.047 percent receive technology-assisted care.

While the proportion of severely afflicted children is relatively low, public and private health care costs for children with special needs are substantial (Ireys et al., 1997; Silber et al., 1999; United States General Accounting Office, 2000). For example, in fiscal year 1998, the 1 million disabled children on Medicaid constituted 7 percent of beneficiaries under the age of 21, but accounted for 27 percent of the $26 billion in payments for children (United States General Accounting Office, 2000).

Improvability and Inclusiveness

The process of developing, implementing, and monitoring a care plan that involves the active participation of the family and health professionals is the most effective vehicle for ensuring comprehensive, culturally sensitive, patient/family-centered care for this population. Developing a care plan using a collaborative, interactive process is important to help families gain an adequate understanding of their child's chronic illness. Even when families play a central role in caring for their child, they often lack an adequate understanding of the condition (Carraccio et al., 1998). Increasing the parents' (and patient's) understanding through educational interventions has been shown to be beneficial (Bauman et al., 1997). Examples of successful interventions include programs for self-management of asthma (Clark et al., 1984), for children with cancer reentering school (Nolan et al., 1987), and for support for parents performing care coordination (Stein, 1983).

Care coordination should help the family obtain the necessary services and ensure that information is shared among all providers and agencies. The care plan should identify specific individuals responsible for coordinating services; all children with special needs benefit from such coordination. A parent, physician, nurse, social worker, school health professional, other medical home staff member, employee of a community-based service, or other support person (such as a family friend or clergy member) can potentially play a significant role in care coordination. School health providers should be included in developing the care plan because about half of children with special needs who require emergency admission to an intensive care unit (ICU) are of school age

(Dosa et al., 2001).

It is also important to note that special-needs patients and their family members often have or develop behavioral and mental health concerns (Breslau et al., 1982; Coupey and Cohen, 1984; Kronenberger and Thompson, 1992; Lavigne and Faier-Routman, 1993; Wallander et al., 1989). Children with special needs have higher rates of mental health problems compared with otherwise healthy children (Pless and Wadsworth, 1988; Wallander et al., 1988; Weiland et al., 1992), and these problems persist (Pless and Wadsworth, 1988). Unfortunately, these children and families too often do not receive needed mental health services (Ireys, 1981; Kanthor et al., 1974; Stein, 1983).

Children with special health care needs require access to a range of medical services, including primary care, medical subspecialty and surgical specialty services, other ancillary services, and dental care. Services are provided in the home, office, emergency room, and hospital. Home care, which continues to evolve, is a major component of health care delivery that must be integrated into the planning process (Guidelines for home care of infants, children, and adolescents with chronic disease. American Academy of Pediatrics Committee on Children with Disabilities, 1995; Ciota and Singer, 1992; Goldberg et al., 1994). In the office, routine pediatric health maintenance and condition-specific preventive care that addresses the prevention and early diagnosis of disease-related conditions or complications are often quite variable and difficult to track (Liptak et al., 1998). Urgent-care needs may supersede routine health care maintenance.

It is important to prepare families for unavoidable emergencies; this is especially so for families of children with special needs who require technology-assisted care (Emergency Medical Services for Children; Sacchetti et al., 1996). Dosa et al. (2001) report that children with special needs are more than three times more likely to have an unscheduled ICU hospital admission compared with previously

healthy children. Among children with special needs, those who receive technology-assisted care are 373 times more likely to have an unscheduled ICU admission than other children with special needs. Almost one-third of ICU admissions of children with special needs are considered to be potentially preventable. Preventable admissions are more common for children with special needs who do not require technology-assisted care (38 percent) than for those who require such care (19 percent). Of preventable admissions, 56 percent are due to the physical or social environment and decisions made by the family.

There is a evidence that improved comprehensive medical care that integrates primary and specialty care has an impact on outcomes (Broyles et al., 2000; Reogowski J., 1998). Broyles et al. (2000) report that comprehensive care for infants of very low birth weight results in fewer life-threatening illnesses, intensive care admissions, and intensive care days without increasing the mean estimated cost per infant for all care.

Diabetes

Aim

To prevent the progression of diabetes through vigilant, systematic management of patients who are newly diagnosed or at a stage in their disease prior to the development of major complications.

Rationale for Inclusion

Impact

Diabetes ranks as the fifth leading cause of death in the United States, affecting 17 million people and a contributing factor to over 210,000 deaths in 1999. In 1997, the total annual economic costs attributed to diabetes-related illness was $98 billion. Of this total, $44 billion was direct costs, such as personal health care spending and hospital care, and $54 billion was indirect costs, including disability, premature mortality, and work-loss days (American Diabetes Association, 2002).

Diabetes predisposes individuals to many long-term, serious medical complications, including heart disease, stroke, hypertension, blindness, kidney disease, neurological disease, and increased risk of lower-limb amputation. For example, diabetics have at least twice the risk of heart disease and stroke of their nondiabetic counterparts (American Diabetes Association, 2002). Diabetes is the leading cause of kidney failure; 33,000 people with diabetes developed kidney failure in 1997. And 12,000–24,000 people go blind each year as a result of the disease (Centers for Disease Control and Prevention, 2000d).

The lifetime cost of complications from diabetes was recently estimated to be about $47,000 per patient over 30 years on average. Management of macrovascular disease is the highest-cost component at 52 percent, followed by nephropathy (21 percent), neuropathy (17 percent), and retinopathy (10 percent) (Caro et al., 2002).

Improvability

Tight glycemic control has been shown to lower health care costs, reduce primary and specialty care visits, and afford short-term gains in quality of life for individuals with diabetes (Testa and Simonson, 1998; Wagner et al., 2001b). In addition, professional and organizational interventions, including aggressive follow-up and patient education, have been shown to contribute to better health outcomes for diabetics (Renders et al., 2001).

The Diabetes Quality Improvement Project (DQIP), a collaborative public–private venture founded in 1997 by the Centers for Medicare and Medicaid Services (CMS), NCQA, and the American Diabetes Association, has developed standardized performance measures for accurately and reliably assessing the quality of diabetes care both within and across health care systems. DQIP measures include, for example, annual testing for HbA1c, annual foot exam and eye exam, biennial lipid testing, and control of blood pressure (Fleming et al., 2001). In a recently published study using DQIP measures to evaluate the quality of diabetes care in the United Sates from 1988 to 1995, it was found that 18.9 percent of participants had high HbA1c values, 58 percent had poor lipid control, 34.3 percent had poor blood pressure control, 36.7 percent did not receive an annual eye exam, and 45.2 percent failed to receive an annual foot exam (Saaddine et al., 2002).

Outcomes from the Diabetes Control and Complications Trial confirmed that lowering blood glucose levels slows or prevents complications arising from type I diabetes. Individuals in the intensive therapy group experienced a 60 percent reduction in risk for eye disease, kidney disease, and neurological disease as compared with the standard treatment group (Implications of the Diabetes Control and Complications Trial, 2002). The lifetime benefits of intensive therapy could translate to approximately 8 years of additional sight, 6 years free from end-stage renal disease, and 6 years' deferral of lower-extremity amputation relative to conventional treatment (Lifetime benefits and costs of intensive therapy as practiced in the diabetes control and complications trial. The Diabetes Control and Complications Trial Research Group, 1996).

The United Kingdom Prospective Diabetes Study analyzed the effect of improved glucose control on type II diabetes. Findings from this longitudinal 14-year study demonstrated a 25 percent decrease in the overall microvascular (retinopathy, nephropathy, and neuropathy) complication rate for patients who received intensive therapy and maintained HbA1c levels at <7 percent. Although no significant effect on cardiovascular complications was observed for lowering of blood glucose levels, an epidemiological analysis did demonstrate a continuous association between the risk of cardiovascular complications and elevated blood glucose levels. For example, a 1 percent point decrease in HbA1c resulted in a 25 percent reduction in diabetes-related deaths (Implications of the United Kingdom Prospective Diabetes Study, 2002; King et al., 1999).

Diabetes is a prime candidate as a priority area because convincing guidelines, a robust set of measures (for example, from DQIP) and known ways of improving delivery of care already exist. Diabetes could serve as a model for improving quality of care for other chronic diseases, particularly with regard to facilitating patient self-management and the active involvement of a multidisciplinary health care team. Improved care for this condition could also stimulate an approach that involves treating other risk factors (cardiovascular disease, hypertension, renal disease) through aggressive management of the disease as opposed to treatment of end-stage complications.

Inclusiveness

During the 1990s, the prevalence of diabetes increased by 33 percent. Most notably, this increase was seen in both males and females, across ethnic groups and educational levels, and among all age groups (Mokdad et al., 2000).

Racial and ethnic disparities have been documented with regard to the treatment of chronic diseases including diabetes (Chin et al., 1998; Institute of Medicine, 2002). For example, one study looking at racial disparities in quality of care for Medicare enrollees found that African Americans with diabetes were less likely than Caucasians to receive eye examinations (Schneider et al., 2002). African Americans are three times more likely than Caucasians to die of diabetes-related causes. And American Indians/Alaska Natives are 2.5 times more likely and Hispanics 1.5 times more likely to die of diabetes than Caucasians or Asians/Pacific Islanders (Centers for Disease Control and Prevention, 2000d).

Box 3-8 Diabetes

The American Diabetes Association recognizes HealthPartners Medical Group of Minnesota as a model for diabetes care. Key components of the HealthPartners diabetes program include a diabetes registry that provides clinicians with automated reminders for needed services; use of interdisciplinary teams including physicians, diabetes nurse specialists, social workers, and mental health professionals; education programs, including counseling on diet and exercise; and implementation of a staged approach to diabetes management, with an action plan and timelines for stepping up care to meet therapy goals. As a result of these multifaceted interventions, improvements in both blood sugar and lipid control were observed over a 1-year period. For example, the proportion of patients with acceptable HbA1c levels (below 8 percent) rose from 60.5 to 68.3 percent, and the proportion of patients with acceptable control of their LDL (bad cholesterol) levels rose from 48.9 to 57.7 percent (HealthPartners, 2000; Sperl-Hillen et al., 2000).

End of Life with Advanced Organ System Failure

Aim

To arrange care so that people facing the end of life with heart, lung, or liver failure will have as few frightening exacerbations as possible, as few symptoms as possible, and as many opportunities for life closure and control of the circumstances of death as possible.

Rationale for selection

Impact

Heart, lung, or liver failure is one of the more common conditions experienced at the end of life (Standards for the diagnosis and care of patients with chronic obstructive pulmonary disease. American Thoracic Society, 1995; Gillum, 1993; Higgins, 1989; Levenson et al., 2000; Lynn et al., 2000; McAlister et al., 2001; Rich, 1997; Rich, 1999; Roth et al., 2000; United States Department of Health and Human Services, 1998). People live with these conditions for long periods of time that have become longer now that better treatments slow the progression of illness. However, the conditions still cause death eventually, and living for a long time in perilous circumstances poses its own challenges. Heart failure is one of the most common hospitalization diagnoses in Medicare, and lung failure is close behind (Standards for the diagnosis and care of patients with chronic obstructive pulmonary disease. American Thoracic Society, 1995; Rich, 1999). As many more people survive their first few heart attacks, their first episodes of lung infection with emphysema, and their first bleeds with cirrhosis, many more live with advanced organ system failure.

The normal course of such conditions is one of stability and comfort on a "usual" day, with a string of those usual days being interrupted by a rather sudden exacerbation in response to some stress (Levenson et al., 2000; Lynn et al., 2000; Roth et al., 2000). A fever, a small new heart attack, or a bowel problem is enough to disturb the fragile balance being enjoyed by the patient (Burns et al., 1997; Chin and Goldman, 1996). Often, one of these exacerbations is the cause of death, but the timing of that eventuality generally remains unclear to within a week of the patient's dying. Good care for this population requires reducing the rate of exacerbations, diminishing their effects, and planning for the eventuality of an unsurvivable episode.

Improvability

Many studies have shown that the rate of exacerbations can usually be cut in half, and sometimes much more (McAlister et al., 2001; Rich, 1997; Rich, 1999). Doing so requires self-care education, reliable availability of medications, early intervention at the least sign of trouble, and mobilizing of services to the home setting. Most important, good care requires continuity in the care plan and in caregivers across time and settings. Some hospice programs support nearly all patients at home at the end of life (Lynn et al., 2000).

Most health care is loosely organized by referral patterns, and patients from the same neighborhood may go to disparate providers. In end-of-life care for persons facing organ system failure, services are probably best organized so that the same provider of services takes care of all persons in one area, or at least so that only a very small number of providers are working in one area. The number of persons affected by advanced heart, lung, and liver disease is not large, so even urban areas cannot efficiently support more than a few services for around-the-clock availability.

Improving care for this population also requires close monitoring and rapid responses. When a patient becomes quite ill, mobilizing of services–including both urgent and end-of-life services–to the home is essential. Thus, implementing good care for this population requires learning how to work in communities, how to plan ahead, and how to provide good care for very sick people in their homes and nursing homes.

Inclusiveness

Heart, lung, and liver failures account for about one-fifth of all fatal illness in the United States (Lunney et al., 2002), and they strike rather equitably across all genders, ethnic groups, and geographic areas. Cirrhosis tends to kill somewhat earlier than the other conditions, with many deaths occurring before Medicare eligibility (Roth et al., 2000). Heart and lung failures tend to reach life-threatening levels in the 65–80 age group (Lunney et al., 2002).

Box 3-9 End of Life with Advanced Organ System Failure:

A Current and Future Scenario

In the current system, an elderly man lives with his wife in a small duplex, and their son lives nearby. As the man has become more disabled with heart attacks and progressive heart failure, his living arrangements have become more constrained. The family moved his bed to the living room, they arranged a long ramp to the door, and they changed the family diet to avoid salt. Nevertheless, he goes into an episode of "failure" every few months and is rushed to the hospital by the emergency ambulance, struggling to breathe. His wife lives in terror of these episodes, and shakes and trembles for days afterwards. She has lived through breast cancer and a stroke herself, and she worries all the time about what would happen to her husband if she died first, and what would happen to her if he died first. Their assets have been spent, and they routinely skimp on their prescription medications, since otherwise they could not meet their rent and food bills. Their son helps out by keeping the place repaired, but he works as a clerk in a convenience store and does not really have funds to assist his parents.

Every time the man is hospitalized, he has a different set of doctors, who never seem even to have his medical record. Between hospitalizations, he is scheduled for a follow-up visit in "resident's clinic," but he does not usually go since it costs so much and seems to do very little good. He does not understand his medications, does not weigh himself, does not know what to do if he starts to become short of breath, and has had no conversations with any physicians in which it was implied that this condition will eventually take his life.

In a transformed health care system, the same elderly man and his wife are enrolled in a complex care management program that ensures that they receive good medical services and helps with financial planning, family support, and advance care planning. Both have come to understand how to manage medicines and weight, and know what extra medications to take at the earliest signs of trouble. The man has had only two more hospitalizations—one for prostate trouble and one for heart failure brought on by a bad cold with a fever. As his condition has worsened, nurses have become available at home. As planned, he eventually dies at home, and the same care team continues to support his wife with the health and living challenges she faces.

Frailty Associated with Old Age

Aim

To arrange care so that people in frail health can count on living in optimally safe environments, free of unnecessary threats to their physical safety, assisted as necessary with the tasks of daily living, encouraged to maintain functioning whenever possible, treated early for complications, and with care shaped by advance care plans that reflect patient and family preferences.

Rationale for Selection

Impact

As Americans routinely no longer die from infections, childbirth, early heart attacks, and the various threats to longevity that were commonplace just a few score years ago, they increasingly live out the end of life in advanced old age, afflicted by multiple medical problems, significant disability, and limiting social challenges, ultimately spiraling into a condition tht can be characterized as frailty (Fried and Walston, 1998; Walston and Fried, 1999). This condition is marked by having multiple chronic ailments and a lack of reserve capacity to endure health setbacks in most body parts and systems (Buchner and Wagner, 1992; Fretwell, 1993; Fried et al., 2001). About half of the people affected past the age of 85 have cognitive deficits from dementia, stroke, or other causes. Many have problems with falls or develop other impediments to mobility. Many have heart or lung problems, but even more have problems with vision, hearing, foot pain, and bowel discomfort (Fried and Guralnik, 1997). Approximately two-fifths of Americans now live with frailty for a few years before dying (Lunney et al., 2002).

The average person living with frailty at the end of life probably faces more than 2 years of self-care disability (Manton, 1989). Unfortunately, the current American health care system was never designed to support large numbers of people with cognitive and other self-care disabilities. Services for frail older adults are often poorly coordinated, entail differing and mismatched sets of eligibility criteria and coverage, and are inadequate to meet important care needs (Moon, 1996; Wagner et al., 1996). The shortcomings have been documented most extensively with regard to nursing facility care, but undoubtedly affect family care at home, paid help at home, hospice care, assisted living settings, and other strategies for services to this population (Bodenheimer, 1999).

The challenge of providing for the large numbers of elderly anticipated over the next quarter century is widely regarded as a major crisis for health care and for society generally (American Medical Association white paper on elderly health. Report of the Council on Scientific Affairs, 1990). Not only will the numbers of dependent elderly nearly double, but also the availability of family caregivers will actually decline.

Improvability

Achieving excellence in care for this vulnerable population will take some time, but some of the needed changes are well documented, highly visible, and strategically important, and it is these changes that the committee recommends making a priority. For example, good care systems have exceedingly low rates of skin breakdown from pressure and poor hygiene. Until the last few weeks of life, when some patients do not want to be turned, the rates can be kept to only a few percent. However, doing so requires assiduous nursing care around the clock (Prevention Program Reduces Incidences of Pressure Ulcers by Up to 87%, 2002; Bates-Jensen, 2001).

As another example, the death of frail patients is no surprise to anyone when it occurs. Advance care planning averts the inappropriate implementation of rescue efforts not desired by patient and family and offering little benefit. In some parts of the country, virtually all persons living in nursing homes or receiving regular home care for frailty have advance care plans that address what is to be done about hospitalization, resuscitation, and other aggressive means to sustain life. In most parts of the country, however, advance care planning is the exception (Fried et al., 2002; Kolarik et al., 2002; Schwartz et al., 2002).

As a final example, many frail people sustain completely preventable injuries due to unsafe home environments. Surveillance of the risks at home, together with the use of improved lighting, warning systems, floor coverings, grip bars, and other environmental modificationsm, has been shown to greatly reduce the incidence of falls and injuries. Yet these measures are not routinely provided or even available to most frail patients (Guideline for the prevention of falls in older persons. American Geriatrics Society, British Geriatrics Society, and American Academy of Orthopaedic Surgeons Panel on Falls Prevention, 2001; Fleming and Pendergast, 1993; Tinetti and Williams, 1998).

In addition, reliable care for the elderly should include interventions such as increased physical activity and strengthening, to prevent further declines in function. For example, in a program designed to prevent functional decline for frail elderly persons, participants were assessed on eight activities of daily living[3] at 3,7, and 12 months, and the results were compared against baseline scores on a disability scale. Moderately frail persons who received the home-based interventions, which consisted of physical therapy targeting improved balance, muscle strength, ability to transfer from one position to another, and mobility, demonstrated less functional decline over time as compared with the control group (Gill et al., 2002).

Improving care for the frail elderly and the provision of support for their family caregivers will require transforming much of health care for this population to a chronic illness model. Continuity and reliability are priorities. Given the large numbers of people involved and the scarcity of caregivers, efficiency needs to be built in from the start. As noted, for example, reducing rates of skin breakdown to the extent possible will require adequate round-the-clock

nursing care, thus pressuring the care system to attend to personal care and not overemphasize procedures. The development of advance care plans for most frail persons will require that professionals learn to counsel patients and families about their future prospects and to maintain effective continuity of the care plan over time. And preventing falls and injuries will necessitate mobilizing services to the places where the frail live, again requiring caregivers to adapt to the needs of this population.

Inclusiveness

Frailty awaits those who survive long enough simply to have diminished reserves, as well as those who encounter mental decline in old age. The condition is now so dominant at the end of life that all ethnic groups, both genders, and all parts of the country are affected roughly equally.

---

[3] Walking, bathing, upper-body and lower-body dressing, transferring from a chair, using the toilet, eating and grooming.

Hypertension

Aim

To reduce the incidence of complications resulting from inadequately treated hypertension (i.e., coronary artery disease, congestive heart failure, renal insufficiency, peripheral vascular disease, and stroke) through early detection, effective treatment, and appropriate follow-up.

Rationale for Selection

Impact

Hypertension (high blood pressure) affects approximately 43 million Americans aged 18 or older, representing 1 in 4 adults. Approximately 20 million of these individuals are not receiving necessary blood pressure medication, and for another 12 million who are being treated, the condition is inadequately controlled (Burt et al., 1995). In 1999, high blood pressure was the primary cause of death for 42,997 Americans and was a contributing cause of death in 227,000 cases. In 2002, the economic costs of hypertension totaled $47.2 billion (American Heart Association, 2001). Table 3-1 presents the estimated number of Americans with high blood pressure by age group.

Overall, 32 percent of people with high blood pressure are unaware they have the disease. If left untreated hypertension can lead to several life-threatening complications, such as stroke, heart attack, heart failure, and kidney failure (American Heart Association, 2002). Table 3-2 shows the extent of awareness of high blood pressure among different racial/ethnic groups.

According to a recent study, the lifetime risk of developing hypertension for middle-aged and elderly individuals is 90 percent.

Table 3-1. Estimated Number of Americans Age 25 and Older by Category of High Blood Pressure

| Age group | Population in Millions | | | |
	Treated, Controlled	Treated, Uncontrolled	Aware, Untreated HBP	With HBP, Unaware
25 – 34	1.7	0.9	1.9	2.9
45 – 64	4.5	4.2	2.8	4.4
65+	3.5	6.9	2.3	5.8

SOURCES: (Burt et al., 1995; Hyman and Pavlik, 2001)

Table 3-2. Extent of Awareness, Treatment, and Control of High Blood Pressure Race/Ethnicity 1988-1994

| Race/ Ethnicity | Percent of Population with High Blood Pressure | | | |
	Treated, Controlled	Treated, Uncontrolled	Aware, Untreated HBP	With HBP, Unaware
Caucasians	24	29	17	31
African Americans	24	32	17	27
Mexican Americans	15	25	19	41

SOURCES: (Burt et al., 1995; Hyman and Pavlik, 2001)

Notably, while women's risk for hypertension remained constant over the two time frames evaluated in this study (1952-1975 and 1976-1998), men's risk increased by 60 percent (Vasan et al., 2002).

Improvability

Data from the Framingham Heart Study and the National Health and Nutrition Examination Survey II indicate that lowering of diastolic blood pressure by a slight percentage–2 millimeters of mercury (mm/Hg) could result in a 17 percent decrease in the prevalence of hypertension, a 6 percent decrease in coronary heart disease, and a 15 percent reduction in stroke (Cook et al., 1995). However, statistics released by the NCQA in its 2002 *State of Health Care Quality* report indicate that of those being treated for hypertension only 55.4 percent maintain their blood pressure at an adequate level. Although this current rate is unacceptable, gains have been made, as the rate was 39 percent in 1999 (National Committee for Quality Assurance, 2002).

A systematic review of 18 long-term randomized controlled trials revealed that the use of low-dose diuretic therapy was effective in reducing stroke, coronary artery disease, congestive heart failure, and total mortality. Additionally, beta blockers were demonstrated to decrease the incidence of congestive heart failure and stoke (Psaty et al., 1997). These findings are consistent with the guidelines of the Sixth Report of the National Committee on Prevention, Detection, Evaluation and Treatment of High Blood Pressure (JNC-VI), which recommends the use of diuretics and/or beta blockers for initial drug therapy for patients with hypertension (The sixth report of the Joint National Committee on prevention, detection, evaluation, and treatment of high blood pressure, 1997). Despite these evidence-based guidelines, a recent study revealed that in 62 percent of visits, physicians failed to introduce proper pharmacologic therapy to patients with a systolic blood pressure of 140 mm/Hg or higher, the JNC-VI recommended cut-off point. On average, physicians were willing to accept a higher cut-off point of 150 mm Hg before believing it necessary to initiate or change drug therapy (Oliveria et al., 2002).

The most recent recommendations of the National High Blood Pressure Education Program Coordinating Committee for primary prevention of hypertension include a two-pronged approach employing population-based strategies and an intensive strategy targeting individuals known to be at high risk, such as African Americans. The recommendations focus on six lifestyle modifications that have not only been proven to be effective in preventing an increase in high blood pressure at the population level, but also can be readily applied to individuals with hypertension or with high normal blood pressure: weight loss; dietary sodium reduction; increased physical activity; moderation of alcohol consumption; potassium supplementation; and modification of diet to include foods rich in fruits, vegetables, and low-fat dairy products and to reduce the intake of saturated and total fat (Whelton et al., 2002).

Inclusiveness

Hypertension affects all races and ethnic groups; however, certain groups are more heavily burdened. For example, compared with Caucasians, African Americans develop high blood pressure earlier in life and have a 1.3 times greater rate of nonfatal stroke, 1.5 times greater rate of heart disease, and 4.2 times greater rate of end-stage renal disease (American Heart Association, 2001). Table 3-3 presents death rates per 100,000 population from high blood pressure by race and sex for African Americans and Caucasians.

Table 3-3. Death Rates per 100,000 Population from High Blood Pressure by Race and Sex

Race/Ethnicity	Death Rates per 100,000 Population by High Blood Pressure	
	Male	Female
Caucasians	12.8	12.8
African Americans	46.8	40.3

SOURCE: (American Heart Association, 2002)

Immunization (Children)

Aim

To sustain the momentum to ensure high levels of immunization coverage for children and to decrease disparities in levels of childhood immunization coverage in metropolitan areas with large populations of low-income residents.

Rationale for Selection

Impact

Vaccines are biological substances that interact with a person's immune system to produce an immune response identical to that caused by the natural infection (United States Department of Health and Human Services, 2000). As a result, they prevent the illness and disability associated with infectious diseases. They also protect society. When vaccination levels are high in communities, the few who are not vaccinated are often indirectly protected because of group immunity. Vaccination is cost-effective as well. Savings range from $2 to $24 for every dollar spent (United States Department of Health and Human Services, 2000). Vaccines in the combined series include diphtheria-tetanus-pertussis or diphtheria-tetanus, poliovirus, a measles-containing vaccine, Haemophilus influenzae type b, and hepatitis B (The Commonwealth Fund, 2002).

U.S. federal and state governments created an immunization system during the 1990s that has demonstrated the capacity to deliver vaccines to children in a variety of health care settings. As a result, record levels of immunization have been achieved across the United States (Institute of Medicine, 2000a). Nonetheless, in 2000 over one-quarter of young children aged 19 to 35 months were not up to date on all recommended doses of vaccines in the combined series (The Commonwealth Fund, 2002). The resurgence of measles in 1989–1991 in the United States was unexpected. Many believe it was fueled by complacency and an absence of data that fostered the mistaken

idea that immunizations were up to date (Institute of Medicine, 2000a). The United States lags behind other nations in achieving widespread vaccination of children (The Commonwealth Fund, 2002). In a study produced by the Partnership for Prevention (2002), vaccinating children is cited as the number one priority among recommended clinical preventive services (Partnership for Prevention, 2002).

Each day sees nearly 11,000 new births, and a strong immunization system is required to ensure the delivery of routine immunizations to these children. In addition to the limited coverage noted above, it is expected that the current system will soon be strained by the addition of new vaccines to the recommended schedule. For example, the American Academy of Pediatrics has recently released a policy statement encouraging that healthy children aged 6-23 months to be immunized for influenza. Recent data has indicated that healthy children younger than 24 months have a high risk of hospitalization due to influenza, and this risk was demonstrated to be greater than healthy adults older than 50 who are routinely recommend to be immunized (American Academy of Pediatrics, 2002; Rennels and Meissner, 2002). Further, state and local budget cuts due to the downturn in the economy are expected to impact the vitality and flexibility of the immunization system. Moreover, studies have noted a strong relationship between low socioeconomic status and vaccine coverage rates (Rodewald et al., 1999). Specifically, children who are poor and live in urban areas may have immunization rates below those in other parts of the United States (Institute of Medicine, 2000a; Rodewald et al., 1999). New strategies need to be developed for reaching out to inner-city populations and raising immunization rates.

Improvability

National objectives include increasing the proportion vaccinated to 80 percent of young children aged 19–35 months (United States Department of Health and Human Services,

2000). Many parents cannot remember the recommended immunization schedule for childhood vaccination, and both parents and providers tend to overestimate the immunization status of their children or patients (Rodewald et al., 1999). Client reminder/recall interventions are strongly recommended by the Centers for Disease Control and Prevention (2000) to remind members of a target population when vaccinations are due. A synthesis of controlled studies revealed that patients who received reminders (such as postcards, letters, or phone calls) about upcoming or overdue immunizations were more likely to be vaccinated or up to date on their vaccinations than those who did not receive such reminders (Centers for Disease Control and Prevention, 2000b; The Commonwealth Fund, 2002).

Multicomponent interventions (including education) are strongly recommended by the Centers for Disease Control and Prevention (2000). For example, vaccination requirements for child care and school attendance can improve coverage and immunity and reduce rates of disease. A decrease in out-of-pocket costs to families for vaccinations and administration of vaccinations has the potential to increase rates of coverage as well; a series of studies showed that this measure led to an improvement in vaccine coverage of 15 percentage points (Centers for Disease Control and Prevention, 2000b).

Inclusiveness

As noted, coverage levels for children less than 3 years of age remain significantly lower among urban and low-income populations (Rodewald et al., 1999). In 1998, 70 percent of children aged 19–35 months from the lowest-income households received the combined series of recommended immunizations, compared with 77 percent of those from higher-income households (United States Department of Health and Human Services, 2000). In California, results of the 1999 California Kindergarten Retrospective Survey indicate that African American and Hispanic children continue to be immunized at lower rates than Caucasians and Asians (Center for Health Improvement, 2001).

Immunization (Adult)

Aim

To increase the proportion of adults who are vaccinated annually against influenza and ever vaccinated against pneumococcal disease through changes in clinical procedures, such as the use of standing orders. Special efforts should be made to improve immunization rates among African American and Hispanic adults and nursing home residents.

Rationale for Selection

Impact

Pneumonia and influenza are the seventh leading cause of death in the United States (The Commonwealth Fund, 2002). Pneumococcal disease causes 10,000 to 14,000 deaths annually; influenza causes an average of 110,000 hospitalizations and 20,000 deaths annually (United States Department of Health and Human Services, 2000). Approximately 30–43 percent of elderly people who have invasive pneumonia will die from the disease (United States Preventive Services Task Force, 1996). The elderly are also at increased risk for complications associated with influenza, and approximately 90 percent of the deaths attributed to the disease are among those aged 65 and older (Vishnu-Priya et al., 2000).

To decrease the burden of these diseases, including incapacitating malaise, doctor visits, hospitalizations, and premature deaths, experts recommend vaccination. Yet one-third to one-half of older adults (aged 65 and over) do not receive these vaccinations (The Commonwealth Fund, 2002). Coverage rates for high-risk adults who suffer from chronic disease are especially poor, with only 26 percent receiving an influenza vaccination and 13 percent a pneumococcal vaccination (Institute of Medicine, 2000). Adults report that they do not get these vaccinations because they are not aware of the need to do so, lack a doctor's recommendation, or forget (United States Department of Health and Human Services, 2000).

Improvability

Adults living in nursing homes are especially susceptible to contagious illness because of close living quarters (Vishnu-Priya et al., 2000). Use of standing orders for immunizations for nursing home residents can improve coverage for this population. Standing orders involve programs in which nonphysician medical personnel prescribe or deliver vaccinations to clients without direct physician involvement at the time of the visit (Centers for Disease Control and Prevention, 2000b). Use of standing orders in settings other than nursing homes has also been shown to improve vaccination coverage among adults. Research has shown standing order programs to result in a median percentage point increase in vaccination coverage of 28 percent (Centers for Disease Control and Prevention, 2000b).

A meta-analysis found organizational change interventions, such as prevention clinics and planned prevention visits, to be highly effective in increasing immunization rates for adults. Specifically, the research focused on strategies that involve searching for system-based problems and solutions and depending on input from teams of involved health care providers to design appropriate interventions (American College of Physicians, 2002).

To increase influenza immunization rates and decrease the possibility of serious illness or death among the elderly, at least 11 states have laws related to immunization in long-term care facilities. For example, New York requires that all long-term care facility residents and employees receive influenza and pneumococcal immunizations (National Conference of State Legislatures).

As noted, the most effective strategies for increasing immunization rates for adults include organizational changes that make the

identification and delivery of immunization a routine part of patient care. Only recently has research been available to identify which such changes work best to improve coverage rates (American College of Physicians, 2002).

Inclusiveness

Both influenza and pneumococcal immunization rates are significantly lower for African American and Hispanic adults than for Caucasian adults (United States Department of Health and Human Services, 2000). The percentage immunized among adults aged 55–64 is lower than that among adults 65 and older, with a median of 38.2 percent nationwide (Institute of Medicine, 2000a). The highest incidence rates of pneumonia are among people over age 65, nursing home residents, and certain ethnic groups, including Native Americans and Alaskan Natives (United States Preventive Services Task Force, 1996).

Ischemic Heart Disease

Aim

To achieve improvements in the prevention of artherosclerotic disease, reduction of reoccurring events, and optimization of functional capacity.

Rationale for Selection

Impact

Ischemic (coronary) heart disease caused 513,758 deaths in 2000, representing 1 of every 5 deaths (Minino and Smith, 2001). The lifetime risk of developing heart disease at age 40 is one in two for men and one in three for women (Lloyd-Jones et al., 1999). Ischemic heart disease plays a major role in physical disability among the U.S. labor force, accounting for 19 percent of allowances by the Social Security Administration (American Heart Association, 2001). Total expenditures for heart disease were approximately $112 billion in 2002, with direct costs, such as hospitals/ nursing homes and prescription drugs, totaling $58 billion and indirect costs, including lost productivity/morbidity, totaling $54 billion (American Heart Association, 2001).

A 50-year retrospective study found that the incidence of heart failure has declined by one-third for women but has remained unchanged for men. However, overall survival rates after the initial onset of heart failure have increased approximately 12 percent per decade since 1950. Despite these gains, heart disease continues to be the leading cause of death among both men and women, with half of patients diagnosed with heart failure in the 1990s dying within 5 years (Levy et al., 2002).

Improvability

A meta-analysis of the effect of lipid-lowering drugs on the incidence of coronary heart disease indicated that drug treatment reduced the risk of nonfatal heart attack and death from coronary artery disease by 30

percent (Pignone et al., 2000). In a study of seven countries, it was shown that an increase in total serum cholesterol was accompanied by an increased risk of coronary heart disease. These findings were consistent across cultures. Notably, however, the absolute level of risk for coronary heart disease was markedly different among cultures, a finding that points to other factors, such as diet, in preventing heart disease (Verschuren et al., 1995). In a randomized controlled study investigating the effect of physical activity on risk factors for cardiovascular disease, it was demonstrated that regular exercise, even with minimal weight change, had a positive impact on lipoprotein levels (Kraus et al., 2002).

Evidence from a retrospective meta-analysis comparing coronary angioplasty and intravenous thrombolytic therapy for acute myocardial infarction (heat attack) indicated that angioplasty significantly reduced the risk of death, repeat heart attack, and stroke. However, it should be noted that lack of access to fully equipped and staffed catheterization laboratories can be an impediment to expeditious receipt of this treatment (Weaver et al., 1997). A recent study examined the cost-effectiveness of early invasive interventions, such as catheterization, for treating acute myocardial infarction as compared with more conservative strategies favoring medical stabilization followed by catheterization for high-risk patients. It was discovered that invasive strategies were more costly by $1600 per patient, but this figure was later reduced to $586 per patient as a result of lower hospitalization rates after 6-month follow-up. Projected estimates of cost of life year gained (between $8,000 and $15,000) supported the use of more invasive strategies, with the exception of low-risk patients (Cohen, 2002; Mahoney et al., 2002).

The use of beta blockers has long been demonstrated as an effective drug therapy for preventing cardiac death following myocardial infarction (Viskin and Barron, 1996; Yusuf et al., 1985). A recent systematic review of randomized controlled trials investigating the use of beta blockers confirmed that these drugs are still successful in reducing mortality and morbidity in patients (Freemantle et al., 1999). However, short-term use of beta blockers after acute myocardial infarction is of questionable benefit unless long-term therapy is sustained.

The Minnesota Heart Survey showed a decline in both out-of-hospital death rates and recurrence of acute myocardial infarction from 1985 to 1997. Marked increases in survival of acute myocardial infarction were also observed. Deaths related to cardiac disease fell 47 percent for men and 51 percent for women. These positive outcomes were attributed to increased use of thrombolytic therapy, emergency angioplasty, angiotensin-converting enzyme (ACE) inhibitors, beta blockers, heparin, and aspirin during this period (McGovern et al., 2001). Over a 20-year period, the Veterans Health Administration in California saw nearly a 10 percent reduction in mortality associated with acute myocardial infarction; 71 percent of this decease was attributed to increased use of aspirin, beta blockers, ACE inhibitors, and reperfusion (Heidenreich and McClellan, 2001).

The Intensive Lifestyle Heart Trial demonstrated that lifestyle changes could slow the progression of coronary artherosclerosis. The intervention group of this study underwent intensive lifestyle changes, including a vegetarian diet emphasizing whole foods with no more than 10 percent fat, aerobic exercise, stress management training, smoking cessation, and group psychological support. In 1 year, a 37 percent reduction in LDL (bad cholesterol) levels and a 91 percent reduction in the frequency of angina attacks were observed. After 5 years, the intervention group showed additional regression of artherosclerosis, whereas the control group showed progression of artherosclerosis and twice as many cardiac events(Ornish et al., 1998). In addition, cardiac rehabilitation, including exercise training, nutritional counseling, and drug therapy, has been shown to reduce morbidity and mortality. However, only 10–20 percent of ideal candidates participate in formal programs (Ades, 2001).

Inclusiveness

Marked regional variations across the United States in the clinical management of acute myocardial infarction have been documented. The Global Utilization of Streptokinase and Tissue Plasminogen Activator for Occluded Coronary Arteries trial (GUSTO-1) found substantial regional variation in the use of both cardiac medications and cardiac procedures. For example, administration of beta blockers ranged from 55 to 81 percent across the country, and angiography from 52 to 81 percent (Pilote et al., 1995). The National Cooperative Cardiovascular Project found that use of beta blockers among patients aged 65 or older varied significantly by state, ranging from 30 to 77 percent (Krumholz et al., 1998; O'Connor et al., 1999). A study examining the treatment of Medicare patients with acute myocardial infarction revealed that a significantly higher proportion of patients received aspirin, IV nitroglycerin, and heparin in urban as compared with rural hospitals. Once again, older patients were less likely to receive recommended therapy (Sheikh and Bullock, 2001).

An evaluation of 81 Veterans Administration acute care hospitals revealed that African Americans were less likely to receive thrombolytic therapy and undergo bypass surgery, even when identified as being at high risk (Petersen et al., 2002). Another study designed to evaluate how race and sex influence physicians' management of chest pain found that women and African Americans were less likely to be referred for cardiac catheterization than men and Caucasians, respectively. In addition, African American women were significantly less likely to be referred for catheterization than Caucasian men (Schulman et al., 1999).

Major Depression

Aim

To improve national rates of diagnosis and appropriate treatment of major depression.

Rationale for Selection

Impact

Major depression is a disorder characterized by depressed mood, loss of interest or pleasure, and other symptoms that may include changes in sleep and appetite and thoughts of suicide. The disorder differs both quantitatively and qualitatively from normal sadness and bereavement (American Psychiatric Association, 1994). Approximately one in seven men and one in four women will have an episode of major depression at some point during their lives (Blazer et al., 1994).

Major depression is associated with an enormous clinical and societal burden in the United States. Depressed patients suffer from levels of disability similar to or greater than those associated with a host of other chronic medical conditions (Wells et al., 1989). The 2000 Global Burden of Disease Study estimates that major depression contributes to more disability in the United States than any other single medical condition (World Health Organization, 2000). Despite this high burden, fewer than half of individuals with depression in the community and in primary care medical settings are correctly diagnosed (Hirschfeld et al., 1997; Simon et al., 1999), and fewer than one-third receive care that is concordant with clinical treatment guidelines (Wang et al., 2000; Young et al., 2001). Rates of treatment for depression are substantially lower than for many other chronic conditions (Druss et al., 2001a), and national health expenditures for depression, while substantial, are low relative to the disorder's associated disability (Druss et al., 2002).

Improvability

A variety of highly efficacious clinical treatments exist for depression, most of which involve psychotherapy, psychopharmacology, or a combination of the two (United States Public Health Service, 1999). Guidelines have been developed for the treatment of depression in primary care (Depression Guideline Panel, 1993; Schulberg et al., 1998), and algorithms are being formulated to guide depression care in specialty mental health settings (Crismon et al., 1999; STAR*D Program, 2002).

Systems of care can be improved to provide better care for depression. A number of interventions have shown that collaborative models designed to improve coordination and follow-up by a multidisciplinary team can improve the process and clinical outcomes of care (Katon et al., 1995; Simon et al., 2000). These models are grounded in principles drawn from Wagner's Chronic Care Model for improving the care of individuals with serious mental illnesses (Wagner et al., 2001c). See Chapter 1 for a discussion of the Chronic Care Model.

Treatment for major depression is increasingly occurring in two settings–primary care medical settings and specialty organizations, which provide services for mental health separately from those for general health care (Frank et al., 1996). Because depression commonly occurs in conjunction with other mental disorders, primary care clinicians are often the first-line providers for the condition's diagnosis and treatment. This practice has become more widespread, with the growing expectation that primary care providers will manage rather than refer common mental disorders, as newer antidepressants are developed that are easier and safer to prescribe (Pincus et al., 1998). With regard to the use of specialty organizations, it has been estimated that approximately 160 million Americans are enrolled in such plans. However, little is known about the impact of these plans on patients' mental health care, and even less is known about their impact on the quality and costs of general medical care for patients enrolled in the programs (Sturm, 1999).

An issue cutting across both types of settings is the fact that mental health benefits are subject to restrictions, such as caps and copayments, not imposed for other medical conditions. A major focus of mental health policy at both the federal and state levels over the past decade has been on seeking to pass legislation mandating parity with general medical benefits. However, the same factors that drive these disparities–economic forces and stigma–may mean that such legislation alone may not be enough to ensure equal access to mental health care (Frank et al., 2001). To truly transform care for depression in the United States, it will be important to monitor not only benefit packages, but also access to and quality of care for depressed individuals receiving those benefits.

Inclusiveness

A number of subgroups may be vulnerable to undertreatment and poor quality of care for depression. Ethnic minorities, older patients, and less-educated patients are less likely to receive antidepressant treatment and more likely to receive lower quality of care than are other depressed patients (Melfi et al., 2000; Young et al., 2001). Minority groups may derive particular benefit from quality improvement in care for depression that can help reduce these treatment disparities (Miranda et al., 2002).

Box 3-10 Major Depression

Partners in Care was a multisite quality improvement project designed to examine whether and how system change could improve care for depression in real-world settings (Wells, 2002b; Wells et al., 2000). The study team worked with leading depression researchers to develop a "toolkit" of services for local primary care providers and patients. This package included an institutional commitment to quality improvement, training in how to provide clinician and patient education, and access to local expertise in psychotherapy or medication follow-up. The study randomly assigned 46 clinics treating 1,356 patients to either this quality improvement program or usual care.

The study found that patients treated under the enhanced systems of care received higher-quality depression treatment, had a better chance of recovering from the disorder, and were more likely to stay in their jobs than those treated in the usual manner. The enhanced care was cost-effective compared with other interventions–an approximately $500 expenditure per patient led to the equivalent of a full month of feeling completely well (over the 2-year follow-up period) and an additional month of employment (Schoenbaum et al., 2001). The Partners in Care study demonstrates that changing systems of care can have a real and profound impact on the clinical care and lives of people with depression, and can do so at a modest cost.

Medication Management

Aim

To prevent and provide ongoing surveillance of adverse drug events (ADEs), and to reduce inappropriate antibiotic use in particular for acute respiratory infections.

Rationale for Selection

Impact

A recent report of the Institute of Medicine placed patient safety issues on the national radar screen by reporting that an estimated 44,000 to 98,000 Americans die each year as a result of medical errors (Institute of Medicine, 2000b). Most common are medication-related errors, which have been estimated to account for over 7,000 deaths annually (Leape et al., 1991; Phillips et al., 1998). ADEs have been associated with longer hospital stays, higher costs, and almost twice the risk of death (Classen et al., 1997). The Adverse Drug Event Prevention Study Group found that ADEs occur in 6.5 of every 100 hospital admissions, with 42 percent of these events being either serious or life threatening (Bates et al., 1995). In another study by the same group, it was determined that the estimated cost for an ADE was approximately $2,600, translating to $5.6 million in annual costs for an average-sized teaching hospital (Bates et al., 1997). Overall, the cost of drug-related deaths and complications exceeds $136 billion a year in the United States (Johnson and Bootman, 1995).

With regard to inappropriate antibiotic use, treatment of acute respiratory infections accounts for 75 percent of all antibiotics prescribed in ambulatory settings. Although the majority of these illnesses are viral in nature and do not benefit from antimicrobial drug therapy, antibiotics are prescribed during over 50 percent of visits for colds and upper respiratory tract infections in the United States annually (Gonzales et al., 1999; Gonzales et al., 1997; McCaig and Hughes, 1995; Schappert, 1997). Such overuse of antibiotics has contributed to

the emergence and spread of antibiotic-resistant bacteria (Kunin, 1993). For example, during the past 5 years, the rate of penicillin-resistant *S. pneumoniea,* the causative agent of pneumonia, has increased by more than 300 percent (Centers for Disease Control and Prevention, 2002a). In a recent study that examined the impact of patient pressure on physicians' prescribing behavior, it was found that in 68 percent cases of acute respiratory infection, antibiotics were prescribed even though 80 percent of those prescriptions were deemed unnecessary according to the guidelines of the Center for Disease Control and Prevention (CDC) (Scott et al., 2001).

The emergence of antibiotic-resistant bacterial strains capable of causing infection alters the initial selection of antibiotics for patients suspected of having a serious bacterial infection. For example, meningitis must be treated with multiple antibiotics that will cover possible resistant bacteria. Not only is this approach expensive, but it also promotes the emergence of bacterial strains resistant to currently effective antibiotics.

Improvability

After assessing ADEs for their root cause, Classen et. al (1998) found that half of the events were potentially preventable. These events included excessive dosage (42 percent), drug interactions (4.6 percent), cases of known drug allergies (1.5 percent), and patient identification errors (3.5 percent) (Classen, 1998; Evans et al., 1992). From 1993 to 1998, the Food and Drug Administration's Adverse Event Reporting System showed that the most common types of fatal errors included improper dose (41 percent), use of the wrong drug (16 percent), and use of the wrong route of administration (10 percent). These errors were attributed mainly to preventable performance and knowledge deficits (44 percent) and communication errors (16 percent) (Phillips et al., 2001).

Computerized physician order entry is a tool that has been shown to reduce medication errors. In one study, use of computer systems equipped with only basic decision support led to a 64 percent reduction in medication errors, and use of systems equipped with advanced decision support resulted in an 83 percent decrease (Bates et al., 1999). Employing a multidisciplinary team approach, the medical intensive care unit at Massachusetts General Hospital in Boston included a pharmacist on its patient care team, which resulted in a 77 percent reduction in medication errors (Cullen, 1998). Barnes-Jewish Hospital in St. Louis has implemented two automated safety net computer systems that detect potentially dangerous drug combinations (PharmADE) and identify inappropriate dosages (DoseChecker). PharmADE has reduced the number of patients receiving dangerous drug combinations at discharge from 36 to 7 percent. In addition, physicians adjusted their original dosage on medications 71 percent of the time after having been notified by pharmacists using DoseChecker (McMullin et al., 1998).

With regard to antibiotic overuse, several studies have demonstrated the positive impact of educational interventions targeted at both physicians and parents to curb inappropriate prescribing of antibiotics. A randomized controlled trial of 12 practices in Massachusetts and Washington State showed that educational outreach to providers and parents resulted in a 16 percent decrease in antibiotic dispensing for children under 3 years of age and a 12 percent decrease for children aged 3 to 6 years. The physician/practice group interventions included two meetings of the group with a physician peer leader who promoted CDC guidelines and feedback on prescribing rates. Parental interventions included mailings of CDC brochures and literature made available in the physician's office (Finkelstein et al., 2001). A community-based intervention trial in Wisconsin designed to enhance awareness of antibiotic resistance and appropriate antibiotic prescribing revealed an increase of 15 percent in parent's awareness after educational interventions and declining expectations for antibiotics for their children (Trepka et al., 2001). In a community-wide campaign based in Tennessee, educational efforts directed at health care professionals, parents, and the general public reduced prescription rates by 11 percent (Perz et al., 2002).

Antimicrobial prescribing rates for children and adolescents have begun to show significant improvement. For example, from 1980 to 1992, a 48 percent increase in antibiotic prescriptions for children was observed as compared with recent data showing a 40 percent decrease from 1989–1990 through 1999–2000 (McCaig et al., 2002; McCaig and Hughes, 1995). Despite these encouraging outcomes, efforts to sustain this downward trend are still essential, as resistant strains of bacteria have continued to emerge during this period. Efforts to reduce inappropriate antibiotic use for acute respiratory infections should continue to be directed at both the clinician and patient/family. Systems should be set up to track antibiotic use for various acute respiratory diagnoses, as well as resistance patterns of common respiratory pathogens isolated in local hospitals. This information should be provided to clinicians on a regular basis, and clinicians should as a community set goals for reducing inappropriate antibiotic use.

Inclusiveness

Although medication errors impact all ages, races, and ethnic groups, certain groups are particularly susceptible. These include patients with chronic illness who are being treated with multiple medications. For example, several studies have shown that 14–24 percent of the elderly were inappropriately prescribed drugs that could have been harmful or of questionable value (General Accounting Office, 1995; Leatherman and McCarthy, 2002; Meredith et al., 2001; Spore et al., 1997; Stuck et al., 1994; Willcox et al., 1994; Zhan et al., 2001). Children also have a higher risk of an ADE related to dosing errors because their medications must be adjusted to their weight (Kaushal et al., 2001).

Although the bulk of research on medication errors has been conducted in hospitals, the problem clearly is not isolated to this type of setting. In one study that examined drug complications in 11 ambulatory clinics in Boston, 18 percent of patients reported such a complication, while a chart review revealed only a 3 percent ADE rate. In 13 percent of the cases, the patient had already had a documented reaction to the drug (Gandhi et al., 2000).

With regard to antibiotic overuse, since children and adolescents have the highest rates of antibiotic use and infection with antibiotic-resistant microorganisms, they are a subgroup warranting particular attention (McCaig and Hughes, 1995; Nyquist et al., 1998; Perz et al., 2002; Whitney et al., 2000). The increased distribution of antimicrobial-resistant bacteria also poses a threat to the elderly, who are more vulnerable to nosocomial infections as they are more likely to be hospitalized or in a nursing home (Norman, 2002). Adults, too, are at risk, as they are often treated with antibiotics for viral-related illnesses. In a study comparing antibiotics with placebos for treatment of acute cough in adults, it was found that resolution of the cough was not affected by antibiotic treatment and that the risk of potential antibiotic side effects outweighed any marginal benefit of the drug therapy (Fahey et al., 1998).

Nosocomial Infections

Aim

To significantly reduce the number of preventable nosocomial infections in the nation's hospitals and care centers through the implementation of CDC guidelines (Centers for Disease Control and Prevention, 2000c) and other evidenced-based protocols, coupled with a surveillance system for voluntary monitoring. CDC defines a nosocomial infection as a localized or systemic condition that resulted from an adverse reaction to the presence of an infectious agent(s) or toxin(s) and was not present or incubating at the time of admission to the hospital (Garner et al., 1996).

Rationale for Selection

Impact

Nosocomial infections account for 50 percent of all major hospital complications (Becker et al., 1987). Up to 2 million Americans every year–1 in 20 of all those admitted to hospitals–contract such infections (MMWR Weekly, 2000). In 1995, nosocomial infections cost $4.5 billion and contributed to more than 88,000 deaths, translating to 1 death every 6 minutes (Weinstein, 1998). Nosocomial bloodstream infections are a leading cause of death in the United States, with 57 being the median age of those who die from these infections. It has been estimated that the total number of years of life lost annually in the United States as a result of nosocomial infections is 350,000 (Wenzel and Edmond, 2001).

Improvability

CDC has developed seven guidelines for the prevention of health care–associated infections. These guidelines cover the following: prevention of catheter-associated urinary tract infections, hand washing and hospital environmental control, infection control among hospital personnel, prevention of intravascular infections, isolation precautions in hospitals, prevention of nosocomial pneumonia, and prevention of surgical site infection (Centers for Disease Control and Prevention, 2000c).

In addition to the implementation of evidence-based guidelines, it has been shown that surveillance is an effective tool for curtailing nosocomial infections. The Study on the Efficacy of Nosocomial Infection Control (SENIC), which analyzed over 338,000 patient records across the United States, found that hospitals with the lowest rates of nosocomial infection had implemented rigorous surveillance programs (Gaynes, 1997; Haley et al., 1985).

For example, the National Nosocomial Infections Surveillance System (NNISS), overseen by CDC, was established in 1970 to collect data on hospital-acquired infections. The goal of this initiative was to establish a national database to better understand the epidemiology of nosocomial infections, to track antimicrobial resistance trends, and to provide nosocomial infection rates for use by hospitals as benchmarks for quality improvement efforts. Hospitals voluntarily participate in the NNISS program with the understanding that their identity will be kept confidential (Centers for Disease Control and Prevention, 2001b; 2001d; Gaynes and Solomon, 1996b; Richards et al., 2001). Over 75 percent of hospitals across the United States are now voluntarily submitting their nosocomial infection outcome measures. Currently, the database is being expanded to collect information from nursing homes for the next submission cycle. Many hospitals are electing to forego their anonymity and are releasing their results to the public. Participants in the program have experienced dramatic reductions in rates of infection of the bloodstream and other body sites, including the respiratory and the urinary tracts. From 1990 to 1999, bloodstream infection rates decreased by 44 percent, 31 percent, and 32 percent in medical, surgical, and pediatric intensive care units, respectively (Gaynes et al., 2001).

Despite encouraging outcomes demonstrated by the NNISS, the value of surveillance of nosocomial infections as a quality improvement tool is often overlooked because of both time and cost constraints (Gaynes, 1997). Presently there are no state or federal mandates that require hospitals to publicly report their nosocomial infection rates. As of 2000, 315 hospitals were participating in the NNISS, representing only a small fraction of the 5,810 hospitals in the United States (American Hospital Association, 2001).

Although the importance of actions of individuals, such as hand washing, should not be understated, prevention of nosocomial infections through the implementation of evidence-based guidelines and a surveillance program demonstrates how effective systems interventions can lead to more widespread improvements in quality of care. Collection of national data on nosocomial infections provides a benchmark by which individual hospitals can gauge their performance, thus enabling them to design targeted interventions for problem areas (Gaynes and Solomon, 1996a).

Inclusiveness

Nosocomial infections affect both genders and all ethnic/racial groups. They occur in all American hospitals, but they are not limited to hospitals; they are of equal importance in nursing homes, outpatient facilities, and doctors' offices. Reducing the incidence of these infections will involve the concerted efforts of all health care workers.

Pain Control in Advanced Cancer

Aim

To ensure that patients facing incurable and progressive cancer can count on living without serious pain through to the end of life.

Rationale for Selection

Impact

Cancer is the second leading cause of death in the United States, responsible for one out of every four deaths. Approximately 550,000 Americans will die of cancer in 2002, greater than 1,500 people per day (American Cancer Society, 2002). Many with cancer experience substantial pain throughout the course of their illness and that pain is widely dreaded (Cleeland et al., 1994; Sloan et al., 1999). Cancer related pain affects 20 percent to 50 percent of patients at the time of their diagnosis and during subsequent treatment and 55 percent to 95 percent of those in the advanced stages of their disease (Allard et al., 2001). Living with overwhelming pain is demoralizing, removes dignity and interferes with daily life activities (Cassell, 1992; Ferrell et al., 1991).

Improvability

Various programs have shown that the pain associated with advanced cancer can almost always be controlled to a level that the patient finds tolerable and with acceptable side effects, and that more overwhelming pain can be overcome with sedating levels of relief (Fitzgibbon, 2001). Fewer than 10 percent of cancer patients near death have pain that requires sedation to overcome; through most of the illness, at least 90 percent of patients can be comfortable (e.g., a level of less than 5 on a scale of 0–10) with medications and special procedures (Levy, 1996; Zech et al., 1995). Despite proven guidelines for pain relief, such as the World Health Organization's three-step analgesic ladder, which gradually adjusts the potency of medication as the patient's level of pain increases, pain continues to be undertreated

(Mercadante, 1999; World Health Organization, 1996). The National Cancer Policy Board (Institute of Medicine, 1999; Institute of Medicine, 2001b) and others, including the National Institutes of Health (National Institutes of Health, 2002) and the Joint Commission on Accreditation of Healthcare Organizations (Phillips, 2000), have stated that the major cause of serious pain in cancer is failure to use methods already proven effective.

Often, pain is especially bad around the time patients are transferred from one setting to another (e.g., hospital to nursing home) or in cases of poorly supported home care (Bernabei et al., 1998). Hospice programs have earned a good reputation with regard to pain management, and anesthesiologists have developed a number of special approaches that limit side effects and optimize pain relief (Lynn, 2001). Achieving improvement in this area requires a number of elements that would be useful models for other reforms:

- Skillful use of pain-relieving medications

- Cooperation in protocols across settings of care (Cringles, 2002)

- Advance planning for changes in setting and increases in pain

- Public education to foster a balanced view of the merits of opioid medications (Allard et al., 2001; Dahl et al., 2002)

- Epidemiological surveillance of the population affected to monitor changes over time and to compare the experience of populations defined by geography, delivery system, age, type of cancer, and other factors

Overall, it would be a triumph for the nation to be able to count on competent and reliable pain prevention and relief throughout the course of fatal cancer.

Inclusiveness

While there are small differences in rates of fatal cancer across populations, the disease is commonplace among the rich and the poor, in all parts of the country, and among every ethnic and religious group. African Americans have higher rates of cancer, and die of it both more often and earlier, than Caucasians, Asians, or Hispanics (American Cancer Society, 2002; Hodgson et al., 2001). Some evidence indicates that minorities are less likely to be treated effectively for pain (Anderson et al., 2002).

Box 3-11 Pain Control in Advanced Cancer:

A Current and Future Scenario

In the current system, the Main Street Church support group for advanced cancer patients meets every week, and at this meeting, as at many others, the conversation turns to the reality and the fear of pain. One participant has a doctor who will not give anything very strong yet "because you'll need those strong drugs later." Only when she got her granddaughter, a nurse, to help her change doctors did she become comfortable enough even to come to the support group meetings. Another participant had a problem getting a pharmacy to fill his prescription, and none would deliver it to his part of town, "which was considered too dangerous." A third participant had just come home from the hospital, where he had been in terrible pain for days while the house staff and attending physician made adjustments to his medications on morning rounds each day. It took a week before he became comfortable enough to sleep or eat. Still another participant is not at the meeting, being "too exhausted from not sleeping" since she moved into a nursing home and cannot take her medications when she wants them. The social worker coordinating the support group helps participants deal with their anger and frustration.

In a transformed system, the Main Street Church support group for advanced cancer patients meets every week, and usually the participants discuss family concerns and spiritual issues. One participant mentions that her mother was afraid her daughter would be miserable when she went to the local university hospital for special treatment because her aunt had had that experience 10 years ago. The participant's mother was delighted to find that things had changed and the care was excellent, including asking about and ensuring comfort. Another participant reflects on a conversation with his doctor about his fears that pain might "get out of hand" as his cancer got worse, but his doctor was able to reassure him that this would not occur, citing data from the regional cancer alliance's interviews with patients and family members about their experiences. Two other participants move the conversation along to other topics because there is just not much to say about pain when everyone is confident that it will never be allowed to become overwhelming.

Pregnancy and Childbirth

Aim

To improve the quality of care provided during pregnancy and childbirth by appropriately using proven health-care interventions at key times during pregnancy and delivery, and successfully applying these interventions to populations known to be at risk.

Rationale for selection

Impact

Pregnancy and childbirth may be associated with several complications and adverse outcomes, such as preterm delivery (11 percent), preeclampia (4 percent), gestational diabetes (2-3 percent), and multiple gestations (1 percent), with each of these factors contributing to greater perinatal morbidity and mortality (Martin et al., 2001). In 2000, there were approximately 4 million births in the United States. Of these births, 23 percent were delivered by cesarean section, making this the most common major surgical procedure in the United States (Hoyert et al., 2001).

The annual maternal mortality rate during 1982-1996 remained essentially unchanged at 7.5 maternal deaths per 100,000 live births (Maternal mortality—United States, 1982-1996, 1998), and the infant mortality rate in 2000 was 6.9 per 1000 live births (Hoyert et al., 2001). Many women still miss the opportunity for health promotion and disease prevention early in pregnancy, with approximately 17 percent of mothers not starting prenatal care in the first trimester (Hoyert et al., 2001).

Effective management of pregnancy, including prenatal and intrapartum care, offers opportunities and challenges for quality improvement given the diverse group of conditions and interventions involved, such as infectious diseases (particularly sexually transmitted diseases and HIV/AIDS); chronic diseases (particularly diabetes and hypertension); tobacco cessation counseling;

and management of surgical complications. Moreover, quality improvements in this area could simultaneously enhance health outcomes for two distinct but inextricably interrelated populations–mothers and newborns. Finally, since pregnancy represents a pivotal leverage point for promoting healthy behavior, and since neonatal morbidity will affect a child for many years, health care interventions at this critical juncture can have a lasting impact (Huntington and Connell, 1994; Kogan et al., 1998; Rogowski, 1998).

Improvability

There are multiple opportunities for quality improvement related to prenatal care and intrapartum (labor and delivery) management. A recent study demonstrated that both Caucasian and African American women who received prenatal care experienced fewer neonatal deaths. Lack of prenatal care was associated with higher infant death rates, particularly if complications presented, such as preterm premature rupture of membranes, placenta previa, fetal growth restriction, and post-term pregnancy (Vintzileos et al., 2002).

A recent national survey indicated that only 30-32 percent of physicians screened pregnant women for sexually transmitted diseases. Screening rates were higher among obstetricians/gynecologists and ranged from 75 to 85 percent, however, these rates were still below nationally recommended guidelines (St Lawrence et al., 2002).

Tobacco cessation counseling can serve as the exemplar for this priority area. Smoking during pregnancy has been estimated to cause about 7–10 percent of preterm deliveries, 17–26 percent of low-birth-weight births, and 5–6 percent of perinatal deaths (United States Preventive Services Task Force, 1996). Fortunately, tobacco cessation interventions during early pregnancy have been demonstrated to improve perinatal outcomes, as well as to increase abstinence rates. Data from randomized controlled clinical trials have shown that smoking cessation counseling can reduce the incidence of intrauterine growth retardation and decrease the risk of low-birth-weight births (Law and Tang, 1995; Lumley et al., 2000; United States Preventive Services Task Force, 1996). In addition, tobacco cessation programs have been shown to be cost-effective (Shipp et al., 1992). Despite this evidence supporting their effectiveness, such programs do not appear to have been universally developed and incorporated into prenatal care.

During labor and delivery, specific opportunities for quality improvement include continuing to increase the appropriate use of antenatal corticosteroids (Leviton et al., 1999), decreasing the inappropriate use of tocolytics in threatened preterm labor (Jones et al., 2000), ensuring appropriate antibiotic treatment for preterm premature rupture of membranes (Egarter et al., 1996), reducing rates of inappropriate elective induction of labor (Kozak and Weeks, 2002), and promoting appropriate use of cesarean delivery (Bailit et al., 2002).

Inclusiveness

Pregnancy and childbirth is a priority area that is clearly relevant for a broad range of populations. Women and their families of all demographic profiles are affected by the quality of care provided during the prenatal period and delivery.

Substantial racial/ethnic disparities have been documented for both maternal and infant mortality. Maternal mortality rates are higher for African American women (25 per 100,000 births) and for Hispanic women (10 per 100,000 births) than for Caucasian women (6 per 100,000 births) (Centers for Disease Control and Prevention, 2002c). The infant mortality rate is 2.5 greater for African American than for Caucasian newborns (Beck et al., 2002). The percent of women receiving prenatal care in the first trimester varies by race, with African Americans and Hispanics being 14 percent less likely to receive prenatal care than Caucasians (Hoyert et al., 2001).

Marked geographic variations in prenatal care also exist. In 1999, 16.1-29.9 percent of women who responded to the CDC's Pregnancy Risk Assessment Monitoring System reported having received prenatal care late or not at all. The prevalence of late or no prenatal care was lowest in Maine and highest in Oklahoma (Beck et al., 2002). Variations in the rates of infant mortality have been demonstrated in U.S. metropolitan areas, with postneonatal mortality among American Indians and Alaskan natives being twice that of Caucasians (Grossman et al., 2002).

Severe and Persistent Mental Illness

Aim

To improve care for patients with severe and persistent mental illness treated in the public mental health sector.

Rationale for Selection

Impact

Clinically and legally, severe and persistent mental illness is defined through "diagnosis, disability, and duration" (Senate report number 102-397,). The term encompasses disorders with psychotic symptoms, such as schizophrenia, bipolar disorder, and autism, as well as severe forms of other conditions, such as major depression. From a systems perspective, patients with these conditions are commonly treated in the public mental health sector (Narrow et al., 2000). This sector, which includes state hospitals, community mental health centers, the Veterans Administration, and other state and federal government programs, provides a safety net for individuals who do not have or have exhausted private health insurance benefits.

About 3 percent of the adult population in the United States experiences severe mental disorders in a 1-year period. During 1990, these patients accounted for an estimated $74 billion in national expenditures (Health care reform for Americans with severe mental illnesses: Report of the National Advisory Mental Health Council, 1993). Despite this clinical and financial burden, care for these patients remains inadequate. As many as half of all individuals with severe mental illness receive no care at all (Narrow et al., 2000; Von Korff et al., 1985), most commonly because they do not regard themselves as having a problem that requires treatment (Kessler et al., 2001). Once in treatment, only about a third of individuals with serious mental illness (a somewhat broader group than those with severe mental illness) receive treatment that is concordant with treatment guidelines (Wang et al., 2002).

Improvability

As with other disabling chronic illnesses, the focus of treatment for severe and persistent mental illness is less on curing the condition and more on minimizing symptoms, maximizing function, and preventing relapse. Highly efficacious pharmacological treatments are available to achieve the latter objectives for schizophrenia and other severe mental disorders (Burgess et al., 2001; Thornley et al., 2000; Wahlbeck et al., 2000). Indeed, many of the most important barriers to care for those afflicted with these disorders lie not in an absence of effective treatments, but in the fact that the symptoms and stigma associated with severe mental illness may make it difficult for patients to obtain and follow through with appropriate care. Both case management (Jinnett et al., 2001) and more intensive Program of Assertive Community Treatment programs (described in greater detail below) have been found to be useful means of overcoming these barriers.

Many of the greatest challenges faced by these patients lie at the interface between the public mental health system and other clinical and social service sectors. Much of the best evidence on systems improvability comes from studies of programs seeking to better integrate care across these boundaries. For example, patients with severe mental disorders have been shown to derive substantial benefit from interventions designed to improve the integration of mental health services with substance use treatment (Drake and Mueser, 2000), work rehabilitation (Drake et al., 1999; Lehman et al., 2002), and primary medical health care (Druss et al., 2001b).

The existence of a separate public mental health sector poses a unique set of challenges to efforts to transform the care of patients with severe and persistent mental disorders. First, the presence of this safety net system has made it relatively easy for private insurers to cap lifetime limits on mental health benefits, with the knowledge that patients exceeding those caps will likely be eligible for treatment in the public sector. Similarly, the public system provides a mechanism for private hospitals to engage in "dumping"–the economically motivated transfer of patients into public-sector settings (Schlesinger et al., 1997). The fact that the states bear ultimate responsibility for these sickest of patients has made care inconsistent across states and vulnerable to shortfalls in state budgets. Indeed, state programs face increasing fiscal strain as they seek to care for these patients with limited, and often shrinking, financial resources (Lamb and Bachrach, 2000). Finally, it has been argued that the "two-tiered" (private–public) mental health system perpetuates both the stigma and the social disadvantages experienced by patients treated in the public mental health sector (Hogan, 1998).

One of the best-validated models for improving care for patients with severe mental illness is the Program of Assertive Community Treatment model, or PACT. This service-delivery model provides intensive, community-based services to patients at high risk of psychiatric hospitalization. It was developed during the early 1970s as a response to the deinstiutionalization movement to allow the most severely ill patients to live and function successfully in the community (Marx et al., 1973). In the years since it was developed, it has proved successful in engaging and maintaining these high-risk patients in mental health care, reducing hospital costs, and improving patients' clinical and housing outcomes (Lehman et al., 1997; Marshall and Lockwood, 2000; Rosenheck and Dennis, 2001). Despite these potential benefits, however, only six states have statewide PACT programs, and fewer than half of all states even have pilot programs in place (National Alliance for the Mentally Ill, 2002).

Transforming care for the severely mentally ill will ultimately require transforming the public mental health sector. That transformation will in turn require a federal effort to ensure better standards of care and funding across states, along with a particular focus on interfaces between the public mental health sector, other social service sectors, and the general medical system.

Inclusiveness

The onset of serious mental illness most commonly occurs in early adulthood, and because of their chronic nature, these disorders generally persist throughout the life span. Moreover, they are seen across social classes, ethnic groups, and genders (Tamminga, 1997). Because African Americans with these disorders tend to be overdiagnosed (Baker and Bell, 1999) and undertreated (Dixon et al., 2001; Kuno and Rothbard, 2002), they should be considered a potentially vulnerable subpopulation in treatment studies and quality improvement efforts.

Stroke

Aim

To maximize the stroke patient's abilities and likelihood of returning to a full and independent life.

Rationale for Selection

Impact

Approximately 600,000 Americans suffer from a new or recurrent stroke each year. Stroke is the third leading cause of death in the United States, accounting for 1 of every 14 deaths; in 1999 it was responsible for 167,366 deaths. Stroke is also the leading cause of long-term disability in the United States, resulting in functional limitations and/or trouble with activities of daily living among 1,100,000 American adults. Analyses of the 1994–1995 National Health Interview Survey Disability supplement (NHIS-D) found that among persons aged 70 and older, cerebrovascular disease was the third leading cause of major mobility problems, after arthritis–musculoskeletal conditions and ischemic heart disease (Iezzoni et al., 2001). In 1998, $3.6 billion was paid to Medicare beneficiaries who had short-term hospital visits for stroke (American Heart Association, 2001).

Improvability

A recently published scientific review documents the effectiveness of the following strategies for primary prevention of stroke: adequate blood pressure reduction, treatment of hyperlipidemia, use of antithrombotic therapy in patients with atrial fibrillation, and antiplatelet therapy in patients with heart attack. Additionally, for secondary prevention of stroke, the evidence base supports treatment of hypertension and hyperlipidemia, antithrombotic therapy for patients with atrial fibrillation, antiplatelet therapy, and carotid endarterectomy in patients with coronary artery stenosis (Strauss and Pollack, 2001).

Even the best preventive treatment of stroke does not correct for the inevitable chronic loss of function experience by many patients. Often, this is the area in which the medical system is least effective in dealing with the long-term complications of stroke. In the first few weeks following a stroke, patients may begin to recover spontaneously some of the functional ability lost because of the stroke; this spontaneous recovery may progress for months. Nevertheless, beginning rehabilitation as soon as possible after a stroke can help patients learn better how to accommodate any remaining debility so they can perform daily activities and return home.

Rehabilitation following stroke has been studied extensively, with most researchers agreeing that "a comprehensive, intense rehabilitation program is key to a successful convalescence" for stroke patients (Rosenberg and Popelka, 2000). Therapeutic benefits include better functional abilities, decreased disability, greater likelihood of returning home, and superior quality of life (Cifu and Stewart, 1999; Freburger, 1999; Halar, 1999; Kwakkel et al., 1997; Kwakkel et al., 1999; Rosenberg and Popelka, 2000; van der Lee et al., 1999). To benefit patients maximally, however, rehabilitation must be timely, preferably beginning during acute hospitalization for the stroke, although there is some disagreement about whether more intense treatment improves outcomes (Cifu and Stewart, 1999; Rosenberg and Popelka, 2000). A critical review of 79 studies published from 1950 to 1998 found improved outcomes with better baseline functioning, early intervention, and an interdisciplinary team approach, but no benefit from specialized therapies or greater service intensity (Cifu and Stewart, 1999). One study of over 400 patients revealed that even those without substantial impairment from their stroke benefited from rehabilitation (Roth et al., 1998). The Agency for Health Care Policy and Research (now the Agency for Healthcare Research and Quality) published guidelines for post stroke rehabilitation in 1995 (Post-stroke Rehabilitation Panel, 1995). One medical record review study found that these guidelines are not followed consistently in routine practice (Forbes et al., 1997).

Improvements in this area derive from the seamless integration of care across various settings and clinical disciplines (e.g., medical specialties and/or neurology, physical and occupational therapy, speech–language pathology services). Quality problems are especially likely to occur as patients shift from one care site to another; after a stroke, patients may move several times, ideally to increasingly independent locations. Rehabilitation can occur in a variety of settings, starting with inpatient acute care hospitals and including inpatient rehabilitation hospitals, nursing homes, outpatient offices, and homes. Sometimes Medicare payment policy dictates the location (e.g., restricting payment for nursing homes). Nevertheless, it is critical to ensure that clinicians are monitoring patients' progress over time, tracking functional milestones, and working with patients and their families to make appropriate treatment decisions. Once care moves into the home, oversight of rehabilitation becomes especially challenging. Although physicians must approve therapists' services for the therapists to be reimbursed, many physicians are poorly trained for evaluating and treating functional impairments. The decision about when to stop rehabilitation services is often complex, frequently dictated by reimbursement policies: Medicare generally pays for rehabilitation only when patients are making documented progress toward some prespecified goal.

Inclusiveness

The greatest proportion of stoke-related deaths occurs among those over age 85 (40 percent), followed by those aged 75–84 (34 percent), 65–74 (14 percent), and younger than 65 (11.2 percent). The chance of stroke more than doubles for those above age 55. Stroke is more prevalent overall in men than women; at older ages, however, the incidence in women is higher. Age-adjusted death rates for stroke are 62.4 for men and 60.5 for women (American Heart Association, 2001; Centers for Disease Control and Prevention, 2002b).

African Americans have higher age-adjusted death rates due to stroke than Caucasians–225.2 and 166.7, respectively. Younger African Americans have two to three times the risk of stroke of Caucasians, and African Americans of both genders are more likely to die of a stroke (American Heart Association, 2001; Centers for Disease Control and Prevention, 2002b).

Tobacco Dependence Treatment in Adults

Aim

To improve national rates of screening and appropriate treatment for tobacco use and dependence among adults.

Rationale for Selection

Impact

Tobacco use and dependence represent the nation's single most preventable cause of disease and death. Over 25 percent of adults and over 30 percent of high school seniors–almost 50 million Americans–report regular tobacco use. Tobacco-related deaths number more than 430,000 per year among U.S. adults, including deaths due to heart disease, stroke, lung cancer, and chronic lung disease, accounting for approximately 1 in 5 deaths overall (United States Department of Health and Human Services, 2000). Maternal smoking in pregnancy is the single most important preventable cause of poor pregnancy outcomes, resulting in low birth weight, perinatal mortality, and sudden infant death syndrome (United States Department of Health and Human Services, 2001b). Currently, 27 percent of U.S. children aged 6 and under are exposed to tobacco smoke at home, increasing their risks of respiratory illnesses, middle-ear infections, and decreased lung function (DiFranza and Lew, 1996; Wisborg et al., 1999).

Annual direct medical costs attributable to smoking are estimated at $80 billion–an estimated 6-12 percent of all health care expenditures–not including societal costs due to absenteeism and lost productivity (Max, 2001; The Robert Wood Johnson Foundation, 2001). The direct medical costs of complicated birth are 66 percent higher for pregnant smokers than for pregnant nonsmokers, and the direct medical costs of the effects of parental smoking on children aged 6 and under are estimated at $4.6 billion (Aligne and Stoddard, 1997).

Smoking cessation is extremely cost-effective compared with other preventive interventions (Cromwell et al., 1997). Treating tobacco dependence in pregnancy generates $3–6 in savings for every dollar invested (Marks et al., 1990). On the basis of estimates of both the magnitude of disease and injury prevented and cost-effectiveness (net cost of per quality-adjusted life years saved), assessment and counseling of adults for tobacco use has been ranked the second-highest priority among all 30 clinical preventive services recommended by the U.S. Preventive Services Task Force, and is the single highest-ranked service now in use with less than 50 percent of its target audience (Coffield et al., 2001).

Improvability

Closing the gap between what is known and what is done about treating tobacco use and dependence has been identified as one of the nation's leading opportunities for health care quality improvement (Coffield et al., 2001). Most smokers want to quit, but only about 50 percent of patients report having received smoking cessation advice from their doctor in the past year, and even fewer (25 percent) report any further counseling or pharmacotherapy (Coffield et al., 2001; Thorndike et al., 1998; Tomar et al., 1996). Almost all OB-GYNs report that they ask about tobacco use in pregnancy, but fewer than half go on to discuss cessation strategies and offer self-help materials (The Robert Wood Johnson Foundation, 2002). Healthy smokers are less likely to receive evidence-based smoking treatment than those already suffering from tobacco-related disease (Jaen et al., 1998).

Providers have long reported a lack of training, reimbursement, and supportive office systems as barriers to the delivery of best-practice care for tobacco use and dependence (Glynn et al., 1993). Numerous surveys and reviews have documented limited system supports, insurance coverage, and reimbursement for smoking cessation services (e.g., (Goodwin et al., 2001; Harris et al., 2001; McPhillips-Tangum, 1998; McPhillips-Tangum C, 2001; Partnership for Prevention, 1999;

Solberg et al., 1997). Medicare, for example, provides no coverage for such services (Ossip-Klein et al., 1999). In 2000, only 33 states provided Medicaid coverage for any of the proven treatments recommended by the guideline, and only 21 states covered the no-medication counseling services appropriate for pregnant smokers (Ibrahim et al., 2002).

On the other hand, growing evidence and emerging evidence-based guidelines point to the types of system changes and reimbursement policies that can improve treatment delivery and use. CDC's *Guide to Community Preventive Services* cites strong scientific evidence for recommending multicomponent health care system interventions that include at a minimum a provider reminder system and a provider education program. Such interventions have been found effective in increasing providers' delivery of advice to quit and patients' cessation of tobacco (Centers for Disease Control and Prevention, 2001c). The clinical practice guideline of the U.S. Public Health Service (Fiore et al., 2000) recommends creating clinic screening systems (e.g., expanding the vital signs to include tobacco-use status) or manual or computerized reminder systems as essential to assessment and intervention for routine tobacco use. Both the guideline and the CDC *Guide to Community Preventive Services* recommend reducing patient out-of-pocket costs for effective cessation therapies in light of evidence for increased use of effective therapy and cessation of tobacco use as a result of such measures. These findings fit well with growing evidence that multicomponent system changes (e.g., combining education, performance feedback, reminders, local consensus processes, and incentives) are often needed to promote guideline-based care (Bero et al., 1998) and prevention (Hulscher et al., 1999). The findings are also consistent with a recent review proposing that the organizational and system changes recommended to improve the delivery of preventive care, including treatment for smoking dependence in particular, are fundamentally the same as those recommended by the Chronic Care Model (Wagner et al., 1996) for improving the management of chronic

disease (Glasgow et al., 2001).

Inclusiveness

Americans with the fewest educational and economic resources are most likely to smoke; there are also important variations in tobacco use based on race, ethnicity, and gender (Centers for Disease Control and Prevention, 2001c; United States Department of Health and Human Services, 2000). The percentage of those aged 25 and older with less than 12 years of education who are current smokers is nearly three times that of persons with 16 or more years of education. Overall, American Indians and Alaska Natives and blue-collar workers have the highest rates of adult smoking. Rates of smoking among men (25.7 percent) are slightly higher than among women (21.5 percent). Among Asians and Pacific Islanders, however, rates of smoking are more than four times higher among men than women. Smoking prevalence in pregnancy is at least 12 times higher among women with 9-11 years of education (25 percent) than among women who hold a college degree (2 percent) (Martin et al., 2001), and is particularly common among Caucasian, American Indian, and Hawaiian women. Low-income and minority smokers continue to be the least likely to receive appropriate treatment for their tobacco use and dependence (Fiore et al., 1990; Gilpin et al., 2001).

The harm caused by smoking and the benefits of cessation are apparent across the life span—from maternal smoking and cessation in pregnancy, to the effects of parental smoking/cessation on young children (DiFranza and Lew, 1996; Wisborg et al., 1999), to smoking and cessation among adults 65 and older (Ossip-Klein et al., 1999; Rimer et al., 1990; Taylor et al., 2002). The harm and benefits are also important across the spectrum of health care, from staying healthy, to improving outcomes from acute care (e.g., medication efficacy, wound healing), to improving the management and slowing the progression of chronic disease (United States Department of Health and Human Services, 1990). Besides being declared a chronic disease in its own right (Fiore et al., 2000), smoking is an essential factor in many chronic disease management protocols (e.g., asthma, cancer, diabetes, heart disease).

Box 3-12 Tobacco Dependence Treatment in Adults

Group Health Cooperative (GHC) of Puget Sound undertook a well-documented organizational effort to integrate screening and treatment for tobacco use and dependence into routine health care for all its members. This effort has recently been described with reference to the elements of the Chronic Care Model (Glasgow et al., 2001).

Organizational leadership and incentives were substantial. Senior leaders made reducing tobacco use their top prevention priority. They worked to systematically improve key clinical processes and realign incentives as necessary to achieve this goal; the changes made included supporting dedicated clinic staff, offering incentive to providers, and eliminating patient copayments for smoking cessation counseling (e.g., (Curry et al., 1998; McAfee et al., 1995). *Clinical information systems* were used to create a population-based registry of tobacco users, identified at the time of enrollment and patient visits, to track utilization of cessation treatment resources and to generate patient Quitline calls and provider feedback reports. *Decision support* was provided through extensive provider training, ongoing consultation, and feedback from the automated patient assessment and treatment tracking system. *Practice redesign* and *self-management support* involved the use of a formal treatment program that minimized provider burden by relying on pre-tested self-help materials and telephone counseling to supply essential counseling and pharmacotherapy prescriptions. Finally, linkages to *community resources* included referral to local quit-smoking clinics and related health improvement programs (e.g., weight loss, physical activity, stress management), as well as support for workplace promotional campaigns, smoking restrictions, and other beneficial local policy changes (Thompson, 1996).

Fully implemented in 1993, this initiative has produced a variety of impressive behavioral, clinical, and economic outcomes. For instance, by 1994 the prevalence of tobacco use at GHC had dropped to 15.5 percent from 25 percent in 1985, with comparable data for Washington State showing a much slower rate of decline (McAfee et al., 1995). Rates of tobacco use documentation rose from 40 percent in 1994 to 98 percent in 1999 (Dacey, 2000; McAfee et al., 1995). The proportions of patients enrolled in GHC's formal quitting programs and GHC's overall population quit rate rose substantially with the elimination of copayments (Curry et al., 1998). And compared with continued smokers, quitters who took part in GHC's self-help program used significantly fewer inpatient and outpatient health care services 3 to 5 years after quitting (Wagner et al., 1995).

Obesity

Aim

To improve national rates of screening and appropriate treatment for obesity among children and adults.

Rationale for Selection

Impact

The prevalence of overweight and obesity among Americans has reached epidemic proportions (Mokdad et al., 2001; Yanovski and Yanovski, 2002). The prevalence of obesity has doubled among adults and tripled among children in recent decades, and current trends suggest that prevalence rates will continue to rise (United States Department of Health and Human Services, 2001a). In 1999, an estimated 61 percent of adults (131 million individuals) were classified as either overweight or obese. The prevalence of overweight among children aged 6–11 increased from 4 percent in 1963 to 13 percent in 1999 (the latter figure representing almost 14 million children) (United States Department of Health and Human Services, 2001a).

Over 300,000 deaths are attributed to obesity each year, and experts suggest that the combined effects of sedentary lifestyles and unhealthy food choices that contribute to the development of obesity will eventually make this condition the number one cause of preventable premature death and disability. Obesity is a major risk factor for the leading causes of death and disability: heart disease, including high blood pressure; stroke; some forms of cancer; and diabetes, including insulin resistance and metabolic syndrome (which encompasses some combination of insulin resistance, hypertension, and abdominal obesity and affects an estimated 42 million adults) (Must et al., 1999; United States Department of Health and Human Services, 2001a). Approximately 60 percent of overweight children aged 5–10 already have one associated biochemical or clinical cardiovascular risk

factor, such as hyperlipedemia, elevated blood pressure, or increased insulin levels, and 25 percent have two or more (Freedman et al., 1999). In fact, the obesity epidemic has caused a related epidemic of type II diabetes, including unprecedented rates of type II juvenile diabetes (McGinnis, 2002). In part as a result, obesity now outranks both smoking and drinking in its deleterious effects on health and health care costs, including spending on inpatient and ambulatory care and medication use: adult obesity increases health care costs by 36 percent and medication costs by 77 percent as compared with care for adults of normal weight (Sturm, 2002). Obesity's total costs to the nation are now estimated at $117 billion annually, including $61 billion in direct health care costs and $56 billion in indirect costs (United States Department of Health and Human Services, 2001a).

Improvability

Nearly half of U.S. women and more than a third of U.S. men report having attempted to lose weight, most unsuccessfully (Serdula et al., 1999). Several pharmacological agents, many over-the-counter products, and various diets and dietary weight loss aids and programs are widely promoted but essentially unproven to help Americans combat obesity (Fontanarosa, 1999). However, growing research evidence and emerging evidence-based guidelines indicate the effectiveness of three major forms of treatment for obesity that can be offered through the health care system: counseling and behavioral interventions aimed at lifestyle modification, pharmacotherapy, and surgery (Epstein et al., 2001; National Heart Lung and Blood Institute (NHLBI), 1998; Wadden and Foster, 2000; Yanovski and Yanovski, 2002).

In 1998, the National Institutes of Health published *Clinical Guidelines on the Identification, Evaluation, and Treatment of Overweight and Obesity in Adults,* outlining effective behavioral and medical approaches to the assessment, treatment, and management of overweight and obese patients in primary care settings (National Heart Lung and Blood

Institute (NHLBI), 1998). Behavioral treatments focused on helping people to restrict caloric intake through dietary change and to increase caloric expenditure through greater physical activity can help them lose 5–10 percent of pretreatment weight over a period of 4–12 months, though these weight losses typically are not maintained in the absence of follow-up treatment or environmental changes (Wadden and Foster, 2000; Yanovski and Yanovski, 2002).

Higher-intensity treatments and those that include maintenance components are more successful in promoting sustained weight loss. Current research is exploring innovative maintenance strategies (Jeffery et al., 2000), including those based on the use of information technologies (e.g, telephone, Internet) that can deliver individually tailored interventions in ways that dramatically reduce the counseling burden on busy primary care providers (Boucher et al., 1999). Likewise, there is growing evidence for the effectiveness, health benefit, and cost-effectiveness of individual and family-oriented behavioral treatment for pediatric obesity (Epstein, 1996; Epstein et al., 2001; Goldfield et al., 2001). Pharmacological approaches for treating adult obesity, including recently approved sibutramine and orlistat, used alone and in concert with behavioral treatments, show new promise, as do surgical bariatric treatments, including gastric bypass, for selected morbidly and medically high-risk obese adults (Yanovski and Yanovski, 2002).

Newly released guidelines of the U.S. Preventive Services Task Force recommend intensive dietary behavioral counseling for at-risk adult patients with known risk factors, including obesity, for diet-related disease. The guidelines conclude, however, that there is currently insufficient evidence to support recommending for or against routine behavioral counseling to promote healthy diet or physical activity among general populations of primary care patients (United States Preventive Services Task Force, 2002a; 2003). Recent CDC (2001) data indicate that 58 percent of obese patients received no counseling about weight loss from their health care providers. Another study found that about a fifth of overweight and obese patients did not realize they had the problem–nor did their physicians–indicating that body mass index screening should be made routine (Caccamese et al., 2002).

Inclusiveness

The nation's obesity epidemic has spared no region of the country or segment of the population (Mokdad et al., 2001). Obesity prevalence remains highest, however, among low-income Americans and members of underserved ethnic and racial minority groups. Specifically, the prevalence of obesity is greater among African American, Native American, and Hispanic populations as compared with Caucasians. Behavioral Risk Factor Surveillance System data from 2000 show that the proportion obese varied from 18.5 percent among Caucasians to 29.3 percent among African Americans and 23.4 percent among Hispanics. The contrasts are even greater for women. Among U.S. women aged 18–49, the prevalence of overweight or obesity was 59.9 percent for African American women, 61.7 percent for Mexican American women, and 39 percent for Caucasian women (Centers for Disease Control and Prevention, 2001a). Among children, the prevalence of overweight is increasing more rapidly for African Americans and Hispanics than for Caucasians. Between 1986 and 1998, the prevalence of overweight increased by more than 120 percent among African American and Hispanic children, compared with a 50 percent increase among Caucasians (Strauss and Pollack, 2001).

REFERENCES

Ades, P. A. 2001. Cardiac rehabilitation and secondary prevention of coronary heart disease. *N Engl J Med* 345 (12):892-902.

Administration on Aging. "A Profile of Older Americans: 2001." Online. Available at http://www.aoa.gov/aoa/stats/profile/2001/1.html [accessed July 31, 2002].

Aligne, C. A., and J. J. Stoddard. 1997. Tobacco and children. An economic evaluation of the medical effects of parental smoking. *Arch Pediatr Adolesc Med* 151 (7):648-53.

Allard, P., E. Maunsell, J. Labbe, and M. Dorval. 2001. Educational interventions to improve cancer pain control: A systematic review. *J Palliat Med* 4 (2):191-203.

American Academy of Pediatrics. 2002. "Flu Vaccine Encouraged for Kids 6—23 Months." Online. Available at http://www.aap.org/advocacy/releases/decinfluenza.htm [accessed Dec. 3, 2002].

American Cancer Society. 2001. Guidelines on Screening and Surveillance for the Early Detection of Adenomatous Polyps and Colorectal Cancer. Atlanta, GA: American Cancer Society.

———. 2002. Cancer facts & figures 2002. Atlanta, GA: American Cancer Society.

American College of Physicians. 2002. Annals of Internal Medicine. Pp. 641, 648 *Interventions that Increase Use of Adult Immunization and Cancer Screening Services: A Meta-Analysis.* Philadelphia, PA: American Society of Internal Medicine.

American Diabetes Association. "Facts & Figures: The Impact of Diabetes." Online. Available at http://www.diabetes.org/main/application/commercewf;JSESSIONID_WLCS_DEFAULT http://www.diabetes.org/main/info/facts/impact/default2.jsp [accessed Aug. 6, 2002].

American Heart Association. 2001. *2002 Heart and Stroke Statistical Update.* Dallas, TX: American Heart Association.

American Heart Association. 2002. "High Blood Pressure Statistics." Online. Available at http://www.americanheart.org/presenter.jhtml?identifier=2139 [accessed Aug. 12, 2002].

American Hospital Association. 2001. "Fast Facts on U.S. Hosptials from *Hostipal Statistics.*" Online. Available at www.hospitalconnect.com/aha/resource_center/fastfacts/fast_facts_US_hospitals.html [accessed Sept. 4, 2002].

American Medical Association. "Health Literacy Introductory Kit." Online. Available at http://www.ama-assn.org/ama/pub/printcat/8035.html [accessed Dec. 22, 2002].

American Medical Association white paper on elderly health. Report of the Council on Scientific Affairs. 1990. Arch Intern Med 150 (12):2459-72.

American Psychiatric Association. 1994. *Diagnostic and Statistical Manual of Mental Disorders. 4th edition.* Washington, D.C.:

Anderson, G., and J. R. Knickman. 2001. Changing the chronic care system to meet people's needs. *Health Aff (Millwood)* 20 (6):146-60.

Anderson, G. F. 2002a. *Testimony by Dr. Gerard Anderson, Director of Partnership for Solutions at Johns Hopkins, before the House Ways and Means Health Subcommittee on April 16, 2002.*

———. 2002b. *Powerpoint Presentation: Multiple Chronic Conditions and Functional Limitations.* Presented at May 9-10, 2002 Priority Areas for Quality Improvement Meeting.

Anderson, K. O., S. P. Richman, J. Hurley, G. Palos, V. Valero, T. R. Mendoza, I. Gning, and C. S. Cleeland. 2002. Cancer pain management among underserved minority outpatients: Perceived needs and barriers to optimal control. *Cancer* 94 (8):2295-304.

Anderson, L. M., and D. S. May. 1995. Has the use of cervical, breast, and colorectal cancer screening increased in the United States? *Am J Public Health* 85 (6):840-2.

Antman, Mark. 2002. Personal Communication AMA. Personal communication to Kevin Weiss.

Bailit, J. L., J. M. Garrett, W. C. Miller, M. J. McMahon, and R. C. Cefalo. 2002. Hospital primary cesarean delivery rates and the risk of poor neonatal outcomes. *Am J Obstet Gynecol* 187 (3):721-7.

Baker, F. M., and C. C. Bell. 1999. Issues in the psychiatric treatment of African Americans. *Psychiatr Serv* 50 (3):362-8.

Bastani, R., B. A. Berman, T. R. Belin, L. A. Crane, A. C. Marcus, K. Nasseri, N. Herman-Shipley, S. Bernstein, and C. E. Henneman. 2002. Increasing cervical cancer screening among underserved women in a large urban county health system: Can it be done? What does it take? *Med Care* 40 (10):891-907.

Bates, D. W., D. J. Cullen, N. Laird, L. A. Petersen, S. D. Small, D. Servi, G. Laffel, B. J. Sweitzer, B. F. Shea, and R. Hallisey. 1995. Incidence of adverse drug events and potential adverse drug events. Implications for prevention. ADE Prevention Study Group. *JAMA* 274 (1):29-34.

Bates, D. W., N. Spell, D. J. Cullen, E. Burdick, N. Laird, L. A. Petersen, S. D. Small, B. J. Sweitzer, and L. L. Leape. 1997. The costs of adverse drug events in hospitalized patients. Adverse Drug Events Prevention Study Group. *JAMA* 277 (4):307-11.

Bates, D. W., J. M. Teich, J. Lee, D. Seger, G. J. Kuperman, N. Ma'Luf, D. Boyle, and L. Leape. 1999. The impact of computerized physician order entry on medication error prevention. *J Am Med Inform Assoc* 6 (4):313-21.

Bates-Jensen, B. M. 2001. Quality indicators for prevention and management of pressure ulcers in vulnerable elders. *Ann Intern Med* 135 (8 Pt 2):744-51.

Bauman, L. J., D. Drotar, J. M. Leventhal, E. C. Perrin, and I. B. Pless. 1997. A review of psychosocial interventions for children with chronic health conditions. *Pediatrics* 100 (2 Pt 1):244-51.

Beck, A., J. Scott, P. Williams, B. Robertson, D. Jackson, G. Gade, and P. Cowan. 1997. A randomized trial of group outpatient visits for chronically ill older HMO members: The Cooperative Health Care Clinic. *J Am Geriatr Soc* 45 (5):543-9.

Beck, L. F., B. Morrow, L. E. Lipscomb, C. H. Johnson, M. E. Gaffield, M. Rogers, and B. C. Gilbert. 2002. Prevalence of selected maternal behaviors and experiences. Pregnancy Risk Assessment Monitoring System (PRAMS), 1999. *MMWR Surveill Summ* 51 (2):1-27.

Becker, P. M., L. J. McVey, C. C. Saltz, J. R. Feussner, and H. J. Cohen. 1987. Hospital-acquired complications in a randomized controlled clinical trial of a geriatric consultation team. *JAMA* 257 (17):2313-7.

Bernabei, R., G. Gambassi, K. Lapane, F. Landi, C. Gatsonis, R. Dunlop, L. Lipsitz, K. Steel, and V. Mor. 1998. Management of pain in elderly patients with cancer. SAGE Study Group. Systematic Assessment of Geriatric Drug Use via Epidemiology. *JAMA* 279 (23):1877-82.

Bero, L. A., R. Grilli, J. M. Grimshaw, E. Harvey, A. D. Oxman, and M. A. Thomson. 1998. Closing the gap between research and practice: An overview of systematic reviews of interventions to promote the implementation of research findings. The Cochrane Effective Practice and Organization of Care Review Group. *BMJ* 317 (7156):465-8.

Blazer, D. G., R. C. Kessler, K. A. McGonagle, and M. S. Swartz. 1994. The prevalence and distribution of major depression in a national community sample: The National Comorbidity Survey. *Am J Psychiatry* 151 (7):979-86.

Bodenheimer, T. 1999. Long-term care for frail elderly people—the On Lok model. *N Engl J Med* 341 (17):1324-8.

Bodenheimer, T., K. Lorig, H. Holman, and K. Grumbach. 2002. Patient self-management of chronic disease in primary care. *JAMA* 288 (19):2469-75.

Boucher, J. L., J. D. Schaumann, and N. P. Pronk. 1999. The effectiveness of telephone-based counseling for weight management. *Diab Spectrum* 12:121-23.

Breslau, N., K. S. Staruch, and E. A. Mortimer Jr. 1982. Psychological distress in mothers of disabled children. *Am J Dis Child* 136 (8):682-6.

Brown, M. L., G. F. Riley, N. Schussler, and R. Etzioni. 2002. Estimating health care costs related to cancer treatment from SEER—Medicare data. *Med Care* 40 (8 Suppl):IV-104-17.

Broyles, R. S., J. E. Tyson, E. T. Heyne, R. J. Heyne, J. F. Hickman, M. Swint, S. S. Adams, L. A. West, N. Pomeroy, P. J. Hicks, and C. Ahn. 2000. Comprehensive follow-up care and life-threatening illnesses among high- risk infants: A randomized controlled trial. *JAMA* 284 (16):2070-6.

Buchner, D. M., and E. H. Wagner. 1992. Preventing frail health. *Clin Geriatr Med* 8 (1):1-17.

Burgess, S., J. Geddes, K. Hawton, E. Townsend, K. Jamison, and G. Goodwin. 2001. Lithium for maintenance treatment of mood disorders. *Cochrane Database Syst Rev* (3):CD003013.

Burns, R. B., E. P. McCarthy, M. A. Moskowitz, A. Ash, R. L. Kane, and M. Finch. 1997. Outcomes for older men and women with congestive heart failure. *J Am Geriatr Soc* 45 (3):276-80.

Burt, V. L., P. Whelton, E. J. Roccella, C. Brown, J. A. Cutler, M. Higgins, M. J. Horan, and D. Labarthe. 1995. Prevalence of hypertension in the US adult population. Results from the Third National Health and Nutrition Examination Survey, 1988-1991. *Hypertension* 25 (3):305-13.

Caccamese, S. M., K. Kolodner, and S. M. Wright. 2002. Comparing patient and physician perception of weight status with body mass index. *Am J Med* 112 (8):662-6.

Cadman, D., M. Boyle, P. Szatmari, and D. R. Offord. 1987. Chronic illness, disability, and mental and social well-being: Findings of the Ontario Child Health Study. *Pediatrics* 79 (5):805-13.

Caro, J. J., A. J. Ward, and J. A. O'Brien. 2002. Lifetime costs of complications resulting from type 2 diabetes in the U.S. *Diabetes Care* 25 (3):476-81.

Carraccio, C. L., K. S. Dettmer, M. L. duPont, and A. D. Sacchetti. 1998. Family member knowledge of children's medical problems: The need for universal application of an emergency data set. *Pediatrics* 102 (2 Pt 1):367-70.

Cassell, E. J. 1992. The nature of suffering: Physical, psychological, social, and spiritual aspects. *NLN Publ* (15-2461):1-10.

Center for Health Improvement. 2001. *California Prevention Report: Delivery of High-Yield Clinical Preventive Services by Managed Health Care Plans in California.* Sacramento, CA: CHI.

Centers for Disease Control and Prevention. 1998. *Surveillance for Asthma—United States, 1960-1995.* Vol. 47 (SS-1). Atlanta, GA: MMWR.

———. 1999a. "National Hospital Ambulatory Medical Care Survey (NHAMCS)." Online. Available at http://www.cdc.gov/nchs/about/major/ahcd/nhamcsds.htm [accessed Nov. 13, 2002a].

———. 1999b. "National Hospital Discharge Survey (NHDS)." Online. Available at http://www.cdc.gov/nchs/about/major/hdasd/nhds.htm [accessed Nov. 13, 2002b].

———. 2000a. *Behavioral Risk Factor Surveillance System Survey Data.* Atlanta, GA: U.S. Department of Health and Human Services, Centers for Disease Control and Prevention.

———. 2000b. "Guide to Community Preventive Services (Community Guide)." Online. Available at www.thecommunityguide.org/home_f.html

———. 2000c. "Guidelines & Recommendations: Overview of the 7 CDC Guidelines on Prevention of Healthcare-Associated Infections." Online. Available at www.cdc.gov/ncidod/hip/guide/overview.htm [accessed Aug. 29, 2002c].

———. 2000d. *Unrealized Prevention Opportunities: Reducing the Health and Economic Burden of Chronic Disease.* Atlanta, GA: CDC, National Center for Chronic Disease Prevention and Health Promotion.

———. 2001a. *Behavioral Risk Factor Surveillance System Survey Data.* Atlanta, GA: U.S. Department of Health and Human Services, Centers for Disease Control and Prevention.

———. 2001b. "About NNIS (National Nosocomial Infections Surveillance)." Online. Available at www.cdc.gov/ncidod/hip/nnis/@nnis.htm [accessed Aug. 29, 2002b].

———. 2001c. The Guide to Community Preventive Services: Tobacco Use Prevention and Control. Reviews, recommendations and expert commentary. *Am J Prev Med* (20(2)): Supplement.

———. 2001d. National Nosocomial Infections Surveillance (NNIS) System Report, Data Summary from January 1992-June 2001, Issued August 2001. *Am J Infect Control* 29:404-21.

———. 2002a. *Careful Antibiotic Use: Resistance and Antibiotic Use.*

———. 2002b. State-specific mortality from stroke and distribution of place of death—United States, 1999. *JAMA* 288 (3):309-10.

————. 2002c. "Surveillance and Research Fact Sheet: Increased Risk of Dying from Pregnancy among Hispanic Women in the United States." Online. Available at http://www.cdc.gov/nccdphp/drh/surv_hispwus.htm [accessed Nov. 18, 2002c].

Chin, M. H., and L. Goldman. 1996. Correlates of major complications or death in patients admitted to the hospital with congestive heart failure. *Arch Intern Med* 156 (16):1814-20.

Chin, M. H., J. X. Zhang, and K. Merrell. 1998. Diabetes in the African-American Medicare population. Morbidity, quality of care, and resource utilization. *Diabetes Care* 21 (7):1090-5.

Cifu, D. X., and D. G. Stewart. 1999. Factors affecting functional outcome after stroke: A critical review of rehabilitation interventions. *Arch Phys Med Rehabil* 80 (5 Suppl 1):S35-9.

Ciota, R., and N. Singer. 1992. *Steering Committee on Home Care for Chronically Ill Children, 1987-1992. Final Report.* Syracuse, NY: Central New York Health Systems Agency, Inc.

Clark, C. M., J. E. Fradkin, R. G. Hiss, R. A. Lorenz, F. Vinicor, and E. Warren-Boulton. 2000. Promoting early diagnosis and treatment of type 2 diabetes: The National Diabetes Education Program. *JAMA* 284 (3):363-5.

Clark, N. M., C. H. Feldman, D. Evans, Y. Wasilewski, and M. J. Levison. 1984. Changes in children's school performance as a result of education for family management of asthma. *J Sch Health* 54 (4):143-5.

Classen, D. C. 1998. Adverse drug events and medication errors: The scientific perspective. *Enhancing Patient Safety and Reducing Errors in Health Care.*

Classen, D. C., S. L. Pestotnik, R. S. Evans, J. F. Lloyd, and J. P. Burke. 1997. Adverse drug events in hospitalized patients. Excess length of stay, extra costs, and attributable mortality. *JAMA* 277 (4):301-6.

Cleeland, C. S., R. Gonin, A. K. Hatfield, J. H. Edmonson, R. H. Blum, J. A. Stewart, and K. J. Pandya. 1994. Pain and its treatment in outpatients with metastatic cancer. *N Engl J Med* 330 (9):592-6.

Coffield, A. B., M. V. Maciosek, J. M. McGinnis, J. R. Harris, M. B. Caldwell, S. M. Teutsch, D. Atkins, J. H. Richland, and A. Haddix. 2001. Priorities among recommended clinical preventive services. *Am J Prev Med* 21 (1):1-9.

Cohen, D. J. 2002. Invasive vs conservative management of acute coronary syndromes: Do the data support the guidelines? *JAMA* 288 (15):1905-7.

Cole, S., N. Farber, J. Weiner, M. Sulfaro, A. Silver, and D. Katzelnick. 2002. *Powerpoint Presentation: Depression in Congestive Heart Failure.*

. 2002 *Personal Conversation* Steven Cole.

Cook, N. R., J. Cohen, P. R. Hebert, J. O. Taylor, and C. H. Hennekens. 1995. Implications of small reductions in diastolic blood pressure for primary prevention. *Arch Intern Med* 155 (7):701-9.

Coupey, S. M., and M. I. Cohen. 1984. Special considerations for the health care of adolescents with chronic illnesses. *Pediatr Clin North Am* 31 (1):211-9.

Cringles, M. C. 2002. Developing an integrated care pathway to manage cancer pain across primary, secondary and tertiary care. *Int J Palliat Nurs* 8 (5):247-55.

Crismon, M. L., M. Trivedi, T. A. Pigott, A. J. Rush, R. M. Hirschfeld, D. A. Kahn, C. DeBattista, J. C. Nelson, A. A. Nierenberg, H. A. Sackeim, and M. E. Thase. 1999. The Texas Medication Algorithm Project: Report of the Texas Consensus Conference Panel on Medication Treatment of Major Depressive Disorder. *J Clin Psychiatry* 60 (3):142-56.

Cromwell, J., W. J. Bartosch, M. C. Fiore, V. Hasselblad, and T. Baker. 1997. Cost-effectiveness of the clinical practice recommendations in the AHCPR guideline for smoking cessation. Agency for Health Care Policy and Research. *JAMA* 278 (21):1759-66.

Cullen, D. J. 1998. The effect of pharmacist participation as a member of the patient care team in reducing adverse drug events in a medical intensive care unit. *Enhancing Patient Safety and Reducing Errors in Health Care.*

Curry, S. J., L. C. Grothaus, T. McAfee, and C. Pabiniak. 1998. Use and cost effectiveness of smoking-cessation services under four insurance plans in a health maintenance organization. *N Engl J Med* 339 (10):673-9.

Dacey, S. 2000. Tobacco cessation program implementation-from plans to reality: skill building workshop-group model. *Tob Control* 9 Suppl 1:I30-2.

Dahl, J. L., M. E. Bennett, M. D. Bromley, and D. E. Joranson. 2002. Success of the state pain initiatives: Moving pain management forward. *Cancer Pract* 10 Suppl 1:S9-S13.

Depression Guideline Panel. 1993. *Depression in Primary Care.* Rockville, MD: U.S. Dept. of Health and Human Agencies, Agency for Health Care Policy and Research.

Dewar, M. A., K. Hall, and J. Perchalski. 1992. Cervical cancer screening. Past success and future challenge. *Prim Care* 19 (3):589-606.

Diette, G. B., E. A. Skinner, L. E. Markson, P. Algatt-Bergstrom, T. T. Nguyen, R. D. Clark, and A. W. Wu. 2001. Consistency of care with national guidelines for children with asthma in managed care. *J Pediatr* 138 (1):59-64.

DiFranza, J. R., and R. A. Lew. 1996. Morbidity and mortality in children associated with the use of tobacco products by other people. *Pediatrics* 97 (4):560-8.

Dixon, L., L. Green-Paden, J. Delahanty, A. Lucksted, L. Postrado, and J. Hall. 2001. Variables associated with disparities in treatment of patients with schizophrenia and comorbid mood and anxiety disorders. *Psychiatr Serv* 52 (9):1216-22.

Dosa, N. P., N. M. Boeing, N. Ms, and R. K. Kanter. 2001. Excess risk of severe acute illness in children with chronic health conditions. *Pediatrics* 107 (3):499-504.

Drake, R. E., G. J. McHugo, R. R. Bebout, D. R. Becker, M. Harris, G. R. Bond, and E. Quimby. 1999. A randomized clinical trial of supported employment for inner-city patients with severe mental disorders. *Arch Gen Psychiatry* 56 (7):627-33.

Drake, R. E., and K. T. Mueser. 2000. Psychosocial approaches to dual diagnosis. *Schizophr Bull* 26 (1):105-18.

Druss, B. G., S. C. Marcus, M. Olfson, and H. A. Pincus. 2002. The most expensive medical conditions in America: This nationwide study fund that the most disabling conditions are not necessarily the ones we spend the most to treat. *Health Aff (Millwood)* 21 (4):105-11.

Druss, B. G., S. C. Marcus, M. Olfson, T. Tanielian, L. Elinson, and H. A. Pincus. 2001a. Comparing the national economic burden of five chronic conditions. *Health Aff (Millwood)* 20 (6):233-41.

Druss, B. G., R. M. Rohrbaugh, C. M. Levinson, and R. A. Rosenheck. 2001b. Integrated medical care for patients with serious psychiatric illness: A randomized trial. *Arch Gen Psychiatry* 58 (9):861-8.

Egarter, C., H. Leitich, H. Karas, F. Wieser, P. Husslein, A. Kaider, and M. Schemper. 1996. Antibiotic treatment in preterm premature rupture of membranes and neonatal morbidity: A metaanalysis. *Am J Obstet Gynecol* 174 (2):589-97.

Emergency Medical Services for Children, Task Force on Children with Special Health Care Needs. *EMS for children: Recommendations for coordinating.*

Epstein, L. H. 1996. Family-based behavioural intervention for obese children. *Int J Obes Relat Metab Disord* 20 Suppl 1:S14-21.

Epstein, L. H., J. N. Roemmich, and H. A. Raynor. 2001. Behavioral therapy in the treatment of pediatric obesity. *Pediatr Clin North Am* 48 (4):981-93.

Evans, R. 3rd, P. J. Gergen, H. Mitchell, M. Kattan, C. Kercsmar, E. Crain, J. Anderson, P. Eggleston, F. J. Malveaux, and H. J. Wedner. 1999. A randomized clinical trial to reduce asthma morbidity among inner-city children: Results of the National Cooperative Inner-City Asthma Study. *J Pediatr* 135 (3):332-8.

Evans, R. S., S. L. Pestotnik, D. C. Classen, S. B. Bass, and J. P. Burke. 1992. Prevention of adverse drug events through computerized surveillance. *Proc Annu Symp Comput Appl Med Care* :437-41.

Fahey, T., N. Stocks, and T. Thomas. 1998. Quantitative systematic review of randomised controlled trials comparing antibiotic with placebo for acute cough in adults. *BMJ* 316 (7135):906-10.

Ferrell, B. R., M. Rhiner, M. Z. Cohen, and M. Grant. 1991. Pain as a metaphor for illness. Part I: Impact of cancer pain on family caregivers. *Oncol Nurs Forum* 18 (8):1303-9.

Finkelstein, J. A., R. L. Davis, S. F. Dowell, J. P. Metlay, S. B. Soumerai, S. L. Rifas-Shiman, M. Higham, Z. Miller, I. Miroshnik, A. Pedan, and R. Platt. 2001. Reducing antibiotic use in children: A randomized trial in 12 practices. *Pediatrics* 108 (1):1-7.

Finkelstein, J. A., P. Lozano, K. A. Streiff, K. E. Arduino, C. A. Sisk, E. H. Wagner, K. B. Weiss, and T. S. Inui. 2002. Clinical effectiveness research in managed-care systems: Lessons from the Pediatric Asthma Care PORT. Patient Outcomes Research Team. *Health Serv Res* 37 (3):775-89.

Fiore, M. C., W. C. Bailey, and S. J. Cohen. 2000. *Treating Tobacco Use and Dependence: Clinical Practice Guideline.* Rockville, MD: U. S. Department of Health and Human Services, Public Health Service.

Fiore, M. C., T. E. Novotny, J. P. Pierce, G. A. Giovino, E. J. Hatziandreu, P. A. Newcomb, T. S. Surawicz, and R. M. Davis. 1990. Methods used to quit smoking in the United States. Do cessation programs help? *JAMA* 263 (20):2760-5.

Fitzgibbon, D. R. 2001. Cancer Pain: Management. *Bonica's Management of Pain.* Philadelphia: Lippincott Williams & Wilkins.

Fleming, B. B., S. Greenfield, M. M. Engelgau, L. M. Pogach, S. B. Clauser, and M. A. Parrott. 2001. The Diabetes Quality Improvement Project: Moving science into health policy to gain an edge on the diabetes epidemic. *Diabetes Care* 24 (10):1815-20.

Fleming, B. E., and D. R. Pendergast. 1993. Physical condition, activity pattern, and environment as factors in falls by adult care facility residents. *Arch Phys Med Rehabil* 74 (6):627-30.

Fontanarosa, P. B. 1999. Patients, physicians, and weight control. *JAMA* 282 (16):1581-2.

Forbes, S. A., P. W. Duncan, and M. K. Zimmerman. 1997. Review criteria for stroke rehabilitation outcomes. *Arch Phys Med Rehabil* 78 (10):1112-6.

Frank, R. G., H. H. Goldman, and T. G. McGuire. 2001. Will parity in coverage result in better mental health care? *N Engl J Med* 345 (23):1701-4.

Frank, R. G., H. A. Huskamp, T. G. McGuire, and J. P. Newhouse. 1996. Some economics of mental health 'carve-outs'. *Arch Gen Psychiatry* 53 (10):933-7.

Freburger, J. K. 1999. Analysis of the relationship between the utilization of physical therapy services and outcomes for patients with acute stroke. *Phys Ther* 79 (10):906-18.

Freedman, D. S., W. H. Dietz, S. R. Srinivasan, and G. S. Berenson. 1999. The relation of overweight to cardiovascular risk factors among children and adolescents: The Bogalusa Heart Study. *Pediatrics* 103 (6 Pt 1):1175-82.

Freemantle, N., J. Cleland, P. Young, J. Mason, and J. Harrison. 1999. Beta Blockade after myocardial infarction: Systematic review and meta regression analysis. *BMJ* 318 (7200):1730-7.

Fretwell, M. 1993. Principles of Geriatric Medicine and Gerontology. Pp. 241-8. Vol. Acute Hospital Care for Frail Older Patients, Chapter 22. 3rd edition.McGraw Hill.

Fried, L. P., and J. M. Guralnik. 1997. Disability in older adults: Evidence regarding significance, etiology, and risk. *J Am Geriatr Soc* 45 (1):92-100.

Fried, L. P., C. M. Tangen, J. Walston, A. B. Newman, C. Hirsch, J. Gottdiener, T. Seeman, R. Tracy, W. J. Kop, G. Burke, and M. A. McBurnie. 2001. Frailty in older adults: Evidence for a phenotype. *J Gerontol A Biol Sci Med Sci* 56 (3):M146-56.

Fried, L. P., and J. Walston. 1998. Principles of Geriatric Medicine and Gerontology. Pp. 1387-402. Vol. Frailty and Failure ot Thrive. Chapter 109. 4th edition.McGraw Hill.

Fried, T. R., E. H. Bradley, V. R. Towle, and H. Allore. 2002. Understanding the treatment preferences of seriously ill patients. *N Engl J Med* 346 (14):1061-6.

Gandhi, T. K., H. R. Burstin, E. F. Cook, A. L. Puopolo, J. S. Haas, T. A. Brennan, and D. W. Bates. 2000. Drug complications in outpatients. *J Gen Intern Med* 15 (3):149-54.

Garner, J. S., W. R. Jarvis, T. G. Emori, T. C. Horan, and J. M. Hughes. 1996. CDC definitions for nosocomial infections. Pp. A-1-A-20. Olmsted RN edition. St Louis: Mosby.

Gaynes, R., C. Richards, J. Edwards, T. G. Emori, T. Horan, J. Alonso-Echanove, S. Fridkin, R. Lawton, G. Peavy, and J. Tolson. 2001. Feeding back surveillance data to prevent hospital-acquired infections. *Emerg Infect Dis* 7 (2):295-8.

Gaynes, R. P. 1997. Surveillance of nosocomial infections: A fundamental ingredient for quality. *Infect Control Hosp Epidemiol* 18 (7):475-8.

Gaynes, R. P., and S. Solomon. 1996a. Improving hospital-acquired infection rates: The CDC experience. *Jt Comm J Qual Improv* 22 (7):457-67.

———. 1996b. Interhospital rate comparison issues: The CDC experience. *Jt Comm J Qual Improv* 22 (7):457-67.

General Accounting Office. 1995. *Prescription Drugs and the Elderly: Many Still Receive Potentially Harmful Drugs Despite Recent Improvements*. GAO/HEHS-95-152. Washington, D.C.: U.S. General Accounting Office.

Gibson, P. G., J. Coughlan, A. J. Wilson, M. Abramson, A. Bauman, M. J. Hensley, and E. H. Walters. 2000. Self-management education and regular practitioner review for adults with asthma. *Cochrane Database Syst Rev* (2): CD001117.

Gibson, P. G., H. Powell, J. Coughlan, A. J. Wilson, M. J. Hensley, M. Abramson, A. Bauman, and E. H. Walters. 2002. Limited (information only) patient education programs for adults with asthma (Cochrane Review). *Cochrane Database Syst Rev* (2):CD001005.

Gill, T. M., D. I. Baker, M. Gottschalk, P. N. Peduzzi, H. Allore, and A. Byers. 2002. A program to prevent functional decline in physically frail, elderly persons who live at home. *N Engl J Med* 347 (14):1068-74.

Gillum, R. F. 1993. Epidemiology of heart failure in the United States. *Am Heart J* 126 (4):1042-7.

Gilpin, E. A., S. L. Emery, and A. J. Farkas. 2001. *The California Tobacco Control Program: A decade of progress, results from the California Tobacco Surveys, 1990-1999*. La Jolla, CA: University of California San Diego.

Glasgow, R. E., M. M. Funnell, A. E. Bonomi, C. Davis, V. Beckham, and E. H. Wagner. 2002. Self-management aspects of the improving chronic illness care breakthrough series: Implementation with diabetes and heart failure teams. *Ann Behav Med* 24 (2):80-7.

Glasgow, R. E., C. T. Orleans, and E. H. Wagner. 2001. Does the Chronic Care Model serve also as a template for improving prevention? *Milbank Q* 79 (4):579-612, iv-v.

Glynn, T. J., M. W. Manley, L. I. Solberg, and J. Slade. 1993. Creating and maintaining an optimal medical practice environment for the treatment of nicotine addiction. *Nicotine Addiction: Principles and Management*. C. T. Orleans and J. Slade, eds. New York: Oxford University Press.

Goldberg, A. I., H. G. Gardner, and L. E. Gibson. 1994. Home care: The next frontier of pediatric practice. *J Pediatr* 125 (5 Pt 1):686-90.

Goldfield, G. S., L. H. Epstein, C. K. Kilanowski, R. A. Paluch, and B. Kogut-Bossler. 2001. Cost-effectiveness of group and mixed family-based treatment for childhood obesity. *Int J Obes Relat Metab Disord* 25 (12):1843-9.

Gonzales, R., J. F. Steiner, A. Lum, and P. H. Barrett Jr. 1999. Decreasing antibiotic use in ambulatory practice: Impact of a multidimensional intervention on the treatment of uncomplicated acute bronchitis in adults. *JAMA* 281 (16):1512-9.

Gonzales, R., J. F. Steiner, and M. A. Sande. 1997. Antibiotic prescribing for adults with colds, upper respiratory tract infections, and bronchitis by ambulatory care physicians. *JAMA* 278 (11):901-4.

Goodwin, M. A., S. J. Zyzanski, S. Zronek, M. Ruhe, S. M. Weyer, N. Konrad, D. Esola, and K. C. Stange. 2001. A clinical trial of tailored office systems for preventive service delivery: The Study to Enhance Prevention by Understanding Practice (STEP-UP). *Am J Prev Med* 21 (1):20-8.

Gortmaker, S. L., D. K. Walker, M. Weitzman, and A. M. Sobol. 1990. Chronic conditions, socioeconomic risks, and behavioral problems in children and adolescents. *Pediatrics* 85 (3):267-76.

Grant, E. N., C. S. Lyttle, and K. B. Weiss. 2000. The relation of socioeconomic factors and racial/ethnic differences in US asthma mortality. *Am J Public Health* 90 (12):1923-5.

Greineder, D. K., K. C. Loane, and P. Parks. 1999. A randomized controlled trial of a pediatric asthma outreach program. *J Allergy Clin Immunol* 103 (3 Pt 1):436-40.

Grossman, D. C., L. M. Baldwin, S. Casey, B. Nixon, W. Hollow, and L. G. Hart. 2002. Disparities in infant health among American Indians and Alaska natives in US metropolitan areas. *Pediatrics* 109 (4):627-33.

Guideline for the prevention of falls in older persons. American Geriatrics Society, British Geriatrics Society, and American Academy of Orthopaedic Surgeons Panel on Falls Prevention. 2001. *J Am Geriatr Soc* 49 (5):664-72.

Guidelines for home care of infants, children, and adolescents with chronic disease. American Academy of Pediatrics Committee on Children with Disabilities. 1995. *Pediatrics* 96 (1 Pt 1):161-64.

Halar, E. M. 1999. Management of stroke risk factors during the process of rehabilitation. Secondary stroke prevention. *Phys Med Rehabil Clin N Am* 10 (4):839-56, viii.

Haley, R. W., D. H. Culver, J. W. White, W. M. Morgan, T. G. Emori, V. P. Munn, and T. M. Hooton. 1985. The efficacy of infection surveillance and control programs in preventing nosocomial infections in US hospitals. *Am J Epidemiol* 121 (2):182-205.

Harlan, L. C., A. B. Bernstein, and L. G. Kessler. 1991. Cervical cancer screening: Who is not screened and why? *Am J Public Health* 81 (7):885-90.

Harris, J. R., H. H. Schauffler, A. Milstein, P. Powers, and D. P. Hopkins. 2001. Expanding health insurance coverage for smoking cessation treatments: Experience of the Pacific Business Group on Health. *Am J Health Promot* 15 (5):350-6.

Hartert, T. V., A. Togias, B. G. Mellen, E. F. Mitchel, M. S. Snowden, and M. R. Griffin. 2000. Underutilization of controller and rescue medications among older adults with asthma requiring hospital care. *J Am Geriatr Soc* 48 (6):651-7.

Health care reform for Americans with severe mental illnesses: Report of the National Advisory Mental Health Council. 1993. *Am J Psychiatry* 150 (10):1447-65.

HealthPartners. 2000. "News Release June 12, 2000: HealthPartners Medical Group Recognized by American Diabetes Association for Quality Diabetes Care." Online [accessed Aug. 26, 2002].

Heidenreich, P. A., and M. McClellan. 2001. Trends in treatment and outcomes for acute myocardial infarction: 1975-1995. *Am J Med* 110 (3):165-74.

Higgins, M. W. 1989. Chronic airways disease in the United States. Trends and determinants. *Chest* 96 (3 Suppl):328S-34S.

Hirschfeld, R. M., M. B. Keller, S. Panico, B. S. Arons, D. Barlow, F. Davidoff, J. Endicott, J. Froom, M. Goldstein, J. M. Gorman, R. G. Marek, T. A. Maurer, R. Meyer, K. Phillips, J. Ross, T. L. Schwenk, S. S. Sharfstein, M. E. Thase, and R. J. Wyatt. 1997. The National Depressive and Manic-Depressive Association consensus statement on the undertreatment of depression. *JAMA* 277 (4):333-40.

Hodgson, D. C., C. S. Fuchs, and J. Z. Ayanian. 2001. Impact of patient and provider characteristics on the treatment and outcomes of colorectal cancer. *J Natl Cancer Inst* 93 (7):501-15.

Hogan, M. F. 1998. The public sector and mental health parity: Time for inclusion. *J Ment Health Policy Econ* 1 (4):189-98.

Hoyert, D. L., M. A. Freedman, D. M. Strobino, and B. Guyer. 2001. Annual summary of vital statistics: 2000. *Pediatrics* 108 (6):1241-55.

Hulscher, M. E., M. Wensing, R. P. Grol, T. van der Weijden, and C. van Weel. 1999. Interventions to improve the delivery of preventive services in primary care. *Am J Public Health* 89 (5):737-46.

Hunt, D. L., R. B. Haynes, S. E. Hanna, and K. Smith. 1998. Effects of computer-based clinical decision support systems on physician performance and patient outcomes: A systematic review. *JAMA* 280 (15):1339-46.

Huntington, J., and F. A. Connell. 1994. For every dollar spent—the cost-savings argument for prenatal care. *N Engl J Med* 331 (19):1303-7.

Hyman, D. J., and V. N. Pavlik. 2001. Characteristics of patients with uncontrolled hypertension in the United States. *N Engl J Med* 345 (7):479-86.

Ibrahim, J. K., H. H. Schauffler, D. C. Barker, and C. T. Orleans. 2002. Coverage of tobacco dependence treatments for pregnant women and for children and their parents. *Am J Public Health* 92 (12):1940-2.

Iezzoni, L. I., E. P. McCarthy, R. B. Davis, and H. Siebens. 2001. Mobility difficulties are not only a problem of old age. *J Gen Intern Med* 16 (4):235-43.

Implications of the Diabetes Control and Complications Trial. 2002. *Diabetes Care* 25Suppl 1

Implications of the United Kingdom Prospective Diabetes Study. 2002. *Diabetes Care* 25 Suppl 1:S28-32.

Institute of Medicine. 1999. *Ensuring Quality Cancer Care.* M. Hewitt and J. V. Simone, eds. Washington, D.C.: National Academy Press.

———. 2000a. *Calling the Shots: Immunization Finance Policies and Practices.* Washington, D. C.: National Academy Press.

———. 2000b. *To Err Is Human: Building a Safer Health System.* L. T. Kohn, J. M. Corrigan, and M. S. Donaldson, eds. Washington, D.C: National Academy Press.

———. 2001a. *Crossing the Quality Chasm: A New Health System for the 21st Century.* Washington, D.C.: National Academy Press.

———. 2001b. *Improving Palliative Care for Cancer.* Washington, D.C.: National Academy Press.

———. 2002. *Unequal Treatment: Confronting Racial and Ethnic Disparities in Health Care.* B. S. Smedley, A. Y. Stith, and B. D. Nelson, eds. Washington, D.C.: National Academy Press.

Ireys, H. T. 1981. The Selected Panel on the Promotion of Child Health, Better Health for Our Children: A National Strategy. Pp. 321-53. *Health Care for Chronically Disabled Children and Their Families.* Washington, D.C.: U.S. Government Printing Office.

Ireys, H. T., G. F. Anderson, T. J. Shaffer, and J. M. Neff. 1997. Expenditures for care of children with chronic illnesses enrolled in the Washington State Medicaid program, fiscal year 1993. *Pediatrics* 100 (2 Pt 1):197-204.

Jaen, C. R., B. F. Crabtree, S. J. Zyzanski, M. A. Goodwin, and K. C. Stange. 1998. Making time for tobacco cessation counseling. *J Fam Pract* 46 (5):425-8.

Jeffery, R. W., A. Drewnowski, L. H. Epstein, A. J. Stunkard, G. T. Wilson, R. R. Wing, and D. R. Hill. 2000. Long-term maintenance of weight loss: Current status. *Health Psychol* 19 (1 Suppl):5-16.

Jinnett, K., J. A. Alexander, and E. Ullman. 2001. Case management and quality of life: Assessing treatment and outcomes for clients with chronic and persistent mental illness. *Health Serv Res* 36 (1 Pt 1):61-90.

Johnson, J. A., and J. L. Bootman. 1995. Drug-related morbidity and mortality. A cost-of-illness model. *Arch Intern Med* 155 (18):1949-56.

Joint National Committee on Prevention, Detection Evaluation and Treatment of High Blood Pressure. 1997. 6th report. 2413-46.

Jones, S. C., B. C. Brost, and W. T. Brehm. 2000. Should intravenous tocolysis be considered beyond 34 weeks' gestation? *Am J Obstet Gynecol* 183 (2):356-60.

Kanthor, H., B. Pless, B. Satterwhite, and G. Myers. 1974. Areas of responsibility in the health care of multiply handicapped children. *Pediatrics* 54 (6):779-85.

Katon, W., M. Von Korff, E. Lin, E. Walker, G. E. Simon, T. Bush, P. Robinson, and J. Russo. 1995. Collaborative management to achieve treatment guidelines. Impact on depression in primary care. *JAMA* 273 (13):1026-31.

Kaushal, R., K. N. Barker, and D. W. Bates. 2001. How can information technology improve patient safety and reduce medication errors in children's health care? *Arch Pediatr Adolesc Med* 155 (9):1002-7.

Kessler, R. C., P. A. Berglund, M. L. Bruce, J. R. Koch, E. M. Laska, P. J. Leaf, R. W. Manderscheid, R. A. Rosenheck, E. E. Walters, and P. S. Wang. 2001. The prevalence and correlates of untreated serious mental illness. *Health Serv Res* 36 (6 Pt 1):987-1007.

King, P., I. Peacock, and R. Donnelly. 1999. The UK prospective diabetes study (UKPDS): Clinical and therapeutic implications for type 2 diabetes. *Br J Clin Pharmacol* 48 (5):643-8.

Kogan, M. D., G. R. Alexander, B. W. Jack, and M. C. Allen. 1998. The association between adequacy of prenatal care utilization and subsequent pediatric care utilization in the United States. *Pediatrics* 102 (1 Pt 1):25-30.

Kolarik, R. C., R. M. Arnold, G. S. Fischer, and B. H. Hanusa. 2002. Advance care planning. *J Gen Intern Med* 17 (8):618-24.

Koutsky, L. A., K. A. Ault, C. M. Wheeler, D. R. Brown, E. Barr, F. B. Alvarez, L. M. Chiacchierini, and K. U. Jansen. 2002. A controlled trial of a human papillomavirus type 16 vaccine. *N Engl J Med* 347 (21):1645-51.

Kozak, L. J., and J. D. Weeks. 2002. U.S. trends in obstetric procedures, 1990-2000. *Birth* 29 (3):157-61.

Kraus, W. E., J. A. Houmard, B. D. Duscha, K. J. Knetzger, M. B. Wharton, J. S. McCartney, C. W. Bales, S. Henes, G. P. Samsa, J. D. Otvos, K. R. Kulkarni, and C. A. Slentz. 2002. Effects of the amount and intensity of exercise on plasma lipoproteins. *N Engl J Med* 347 (19):1483-92.

Kronenberger, W. G., and R. J. Thompson Jr. 1992. Medical stress, appraised stress, and the psychological adjustment of mothers of children with myelomeningocele. *J Dev Behav Pediatr* 13 (6):405-11.

Krumholz, H. M., M. J. Radford, Y. Wang, J. Chen, A. Heiat, and T. A. Marciniak. 1998. National use and effectiveness of beta-blockers for the treatment of elderly patients after acute myocardial infarction: National Cooperative Cardiovascular Project. *JAMA* 280 (7):623-9.

Kunin, C. M. 1993. Resistance to antimicrobial drugs—a worldwide calamity. *Ann Intern Med* 118 (7):557-61.

Kuno, E., and A. B. Rothbard. 2002. Racial disparities in antipsychotic prescription patterns for patients with schizophrenia. *Am J Psychiatry* 159 (4):567-72.

Kwakkel, G., R. C. Wagenaar, T. W. Koelman, G. J. Lankhorst, and J. C. Koetsier. 1997. Effects of intensity of rehabilitation after stroke. A research synthesis. *Stroke* 28 (8):1550-6.

Kwakkel, G., R. C. Wagenaar, J. W. Twisk, G. J. Lankhorst, and J. C. Koetsier. 1999. Intensity of leg and arm training after primary middle-cerebral-artery stroke: a randomised trial. *Lancet* 354 (9174):191-6 .

Lamb, H. R., and L. L. Bachrach. 2000. Some perspectives on deinstitutionalization. *Psychiatr Serv* (52):1039-45.

Lavigne, J. V., and J. Faier-Routman. 1993. Correlates of psychological adjustment to pediatric physical disorders: A meta-analytic review and comparison with existing models. *J Dev Behav Pediatr* 14 (2):117-23.

Law, M., and J. L. Tang. 1995. An analysis of the effectiveness of interventions intended to help people stop smoking. *Arch Intern Med* 155 (18):1933-41.

Leape, L. L., T. A. Brennan, N. Laird, A. G. Lawthers, A. R. Localio, B. A. Barnes, L. Hebert, J. P. Newhouse, P. C. Weiler, and H. Hiatt. 1991. The nature of adverse events in hospitalized patients. Results of the Harvard Medical Practice Study II. *N Engl J Med* 324 (6):377-84.

Leatherman, S. and D. McCarthy. 2002. *Quality of Health Care in the United States: A Chartbook.* New York, NY: The Commonwealth Fund.

Legorreta, A. P., J. Christian-Herman, R. D. O'Connor, M. M. Hasan, R. Evans, and K. M. Leung. 1998. Compliance with national asthma management guidelines and specialty care: A health maintenance organization experience. *Arch Intern Med* 158 (5):457-64.

Legorreta, A. P., X. Liu, C. A. Zaher, and D. E. Jatulis. 2000. Variation in managing asthma: Experience at the medical group level in California. *Am J Manag Care* 6 (4):445-53.

Lehman, A. F., L. B. Dixon, E. Kernan, B. R. DeForge, and L. T. Postrado. 1997. A randomized trial of assertive community treatment for homeless persons with severe mental illness. *Arch Gen Psychiatry* 54 (11):1038-43.

Lehman, A. F., R. Goldberg, L. B. Dixon, S. McNary, L. Postrado, A. Hackman, and K. McDonnell. 2002. Improving employment outcomes for persons with severe mental illnesses. *Arch Gen Psychiatry* 59 (2):165-72.

Levenson, J. W., E. P. McCarthy, J. Lynn, R. B. Davis, and R. S. Phillips. 2000. The last six months of life for patients with congestive heart failure. *J Am Geriatr Soc* 48 (5 Suppl):S101-9.

Leviton, L. C., R. L. Goldenberg, C. S. Baker, R. M. Schwartz, M. C. Freda, L. J. Fish, S. P. Cliver, D. J. Rouse, C. Chazotte, I. R. Merkatz, and J. M. Raczynski. 1999. Methods to encourage the use of antenatal corticosteroid therapy for fetal maturation: A randomized controlled trial. *JAMA* 281 (1):46-52.

Levy, D., S. Kenchaiah, M. G. Larson, E. J. Benjamin, M. J. Kupka, K. K. Ho, J. M. Murabito, and R. S. Vasan. 2002. Long-term trends in the incidence of and survival with heart failure. *N Engl J Med* 347 (18):1397-402.

Levy, M. H. 1996. Pharmacologic treatment of cancer pain. *N Engl J Med* 335 (15):1124-32.

Lifetime benefits and costs of intensive therapy as practiced in the diabetes control and complications trial. The Diabetes Control and Complications Trial Research Group. 1996. *JAMA* 276 (17):1409-15.

Liptak, G. S., C. M. Burns, P. W. Davidson, and E. R. McAnarney. 1998. Effects of providing comprehensive ambulatory services to children with chronic conditions. *Arch Pediatr Adolesc Med* 152 (10):1003-8.

Lloyd-Jones, D. M., M. G. Larson, A. Beiser, and D. Levy. 1999. Lifetime risk of developing coronary heart disease. *Lancet* 353 (9147):89-92.

Lumley, J., S. Oliver, and E. Waters. 2000. Interventions for promoting smoking cessation during pregnancy. *Cochrane Database Syst Rev* (2):CD001055.

Lunney, J. R., J. Lynn, and C. Hogan. 2002. Profiles of older medicare decedents. *J Am Geriatr Soc* 50 (6):1108-12.

Lynn, J. 2001. Perspectives on care at the close of life. Serving patients who may die soon and their families: The role of hospice and other services. *JAMA* 285 (7):925-32.

Lynn, J., E. W. Ely, Z. Zhong, K. L. McNiff, N. V. Dawson, A. Connors, N. A. Desbiens, M. Claessens, and E. P. McCarthy. 2000. Living and dying with chronic obstructive pulmonary disease. *J Am Geriatr Soc* 48 (5 Suppl):S91-100.

Lynn, J., J. Lynch-Schuster, and A. Kabcenell. 2000. *Improving Care for End of Life: A Sourcebook for Health Care Managers and Clinicians.* New York: Oxford University Press.

Mahoney, E. M., C. T. Jurkovitz, H. Chu, E. R. Becker, S. Culler, A. S. Kosinski, D. H. Robertson, C. Alexander, S. Nag, J. R. Cook, L. A. Demopoulos, P. M. DiBattiste, C. P. Cannon, and W. S. Weintraub. 2002. Cost and cost-effectiveness of an early invasive vs conservative strategy for the treatment of unstable angina and non-ST-segment elevation myocardial infarction. *JAMA* 288 (15):1851-8.

Manton, K. G. 1989. Epidemiological, demographic, and social correlates of disability among the elderly. *Milbank Q* 67 Suppl 2 Pt 1:13-58.

Marks, J. S., J. P. Koplan, C. J. Hogue, and M. E. Dalmat. 1990. A cost-benefit/cost-effectiveness analysis of smoking cessation for pregnant women. *Am J Prev Med* 6 (5):282-9.

Marshall, M., and A. Lockwood. 2000. Assertive community treatment for people with severe mental disorders. *Cochrane Database Syst Rev* (2):CD001089.

Martin, J. A., B. E. Hamilton, S. J. Ventura, F. Menacker, and M. M. Park. 2001. Births: Final data for 2000. *Natl Vital Stat Rep* 50 (5):11-12.

Marx, A. J., M. A. Test, and L. I. Stein. 1973. Extrohospital management of severe mental illness. Feasibility and effects of social functioning. *Arch Gen Psychiatry* 29 (4):505-11.

Maternal mortality—United States, 1982-1996. 1998. *MMWR Morb Mortal Wkly Rep* 47 (34):705-7.

Max, W. 2001. The financial impact of smoking on health-related costs: A review of the literature. *Am J Health Promot* 15 (5):321-31.

Mayo, P. H., J. Richman, and H. W. Harris. 1990. Results of a program to reduce admissions for adult asthma. *Ann Intern Med* 112 (11):864-71.

McAfee, T., J. Wilson, S. Dacey, N. Sofian, S. Curry, and B. Wagener. 1995. Awakening the sleeping giant: mainstreaming efforts to decrease tobacco use in an HMO. *HMO Pract* 9 (3):138-43.

McAlister, F. A., F. M. Lawson, K. K. Teo, and P. W. Armstrong. 2001. A systematic review of randomized trials of disease management programs in heart failure. *Am J Med* 110 (5):378-84.

McBride, P., H. G. Schrott, M. B. Plane, G. Underbakke, and R. L. Brown. 1998. Primary care practice adherence to National Cholesterol Education Program guidelines for patients with coronary heart disease. *Arch Intern Med* 158 (11):1238-44.

McCaig, L. F., R. E. Besser, and J. M. Hughes. 2002. Trends in antimicrobial prescribing rates for children and adolescents. *JAMA* 287 (23):3096-102.

McCaig, L. F., and J. M. Hughes. 1995. Trends in antimicrobial drug prescribing among office-based physicians in the United States. *JAMA* 273 (3):214-9.

McGinnis, M. 2002. Diabetes and physical activity: Translating evidence into action. *Am J Prev Med* 22:1-2.

McGovern, P. G., D. R. Jacobs Jr, E. Shahar, D. K. Arnett, A. R. Folsom, H. Blackburn, and R. V. Luepker. 2001. Trends in acute coronary heart disease mortality, morbidity, and medical care from 1985 through 1997: The Minnesota Heart Survey. *Circulation* 104 (1):19-24.

McMullin, S T., R. M. Reichley, L. A. Watson, S. A. Steib, M. E. Frisse, and T. C. Bailey. 1998. Experience with advanced technologies that reduce medication errors. *Enhancing Patient Safety and Reducing Errors in Health Care.*

McPherson, M., P. Arango, H. Fox, C. Lauver, M. McManus, P. W. Newacheck, J. M. Perrin, J. P. Shonkoff, and B. Strickland. 1998. A new definition of children with special health care needs. *Pediatrics* 102 (1 Pt 1):137-40.

McPhillips-Tangum, C. 1998. Results from the first annual survey on addressing tobacco in managed care. *Tob Control* 7 Suppl:S11-3.

McPhillips-Tangum C. 2001. *Year 2000 Addressing Tobacco in Managed Care Survey on Health Plans. Paper presented at the 4th Annual Addressing Tobacco in Managed Care Conference.* Nashville, TN.

Melfi, C. A., T. W. Croghan, M. P. Hanna, and R. L. Robinson. 2000. Racial variation in antidepressant treatment in a Medicaid population. *J Clin Psychiatry* 61 (1):16-21.

Mercadante, S. 1999. Pain treatment and outcomes for patients with advanced cancer who receive follow-up care at home. *Cancer* 85 (8):1849-58.

Meredith, S., P. H. Feldman, D. Frey, K. Hall, K. Arnold, N. J. Brown, and W. A. Ray. 2001. Possible medication errors in home healthcare patients. *J Am Geriatr Soc* 49 (6):719-24.

Minino, A. M. and B. L. Smith. 2001. *National Vital Statistics Reports.* Centers for Disease Control and Prevention.

Miranda, J., K. B. Wells, N. Duan, M. Jackson-Triche, I. Lagomasino, and C. D. Sherbourne. 2002. *Can Quality Improvement Interventions Improve Care and Outcomes for Depressed Minorities? Results in a Randomized, Controlled Trial.* Paper presented at the NIMH Mental Health Services Research Conference: July 18-20, 2002.

MMWR Weekly. 2000. *Centers for Disease Control and Prevention - CDC* 49 (8):149-53.

Mokdad, A. H., B. A. Bowman, E. S. Ford, F. Vinicor, J. S. Marks, and J. P. Koplan. 2001. The continuing epidemics of obesity and diabetes in the United States. *JAMA* 286 (10):1195-200.

Mokdad, A. H., E. S. Ford, B. A. Bowman, D. E. Nelson, M. M. Engelgau, F. Vinicor, and J. S. Marks. 2000. Diabetes trends in the U.S.: 1990-1998. *Diabetes Care* 23 (9):1278-83.

Moon, M. 1996. The special health care needs of the elderly. *Baxter Health Policy Rev* 2:317-49.

Must, A., J. Spadano, E. H. Coakley, A. E. Field, G. Colditz, and W. H. Dietz. 1999. The disease burden associated with overweight and obesity. *JAMA* 282 (16):1523-9.

Nadel, M. R., D. K. Blackman, J. A. Shapiro, and L. C. Seeff. 2002. Are people being screened for colorectal cancer as recommended? Results from the National Health Interview Survey. *Prev Med* 35 (3):199-206.

NAEPP Expert Panel Report. 2002. *Guidelines for the Diagnosis and Management of Asthma—Update on Selected Topics.*NHLBI, NIH.

Narrow, W. E., D. A. Regier, G. Norquist, D. S. Rae, C. Kennedy, and B. Arons. 2000. Mental health service use by Americans with severe mental illnesses. *Soc Psychiatry Psychiatr Epidemiol* 35 (4):147-55.

National Alliance for the Mentally Ill. "PACT: Program of Assertive Community Treatment." Online. Available at http://www.nami.org/about/pactfact.html [accessed July, 2002].

National Asthma Education and Prevention Program. 1991. *Guidelines for the Diagnosis and Management of Asthma.* NIH/National Heart, Lung, and Blood Institute.

National Cancer Institute. 1996. "SEER Racial/Ethnic Patterns of Cancer in the United States, 1988-1992." Online. Available at http://seer.cancer.gov/publications/ethnicity/ [accessed Nov. 20, 2002].

National Committee for Quality Assurance. 1997. *HEDIS 3.0. What's In It and Why It Matters.* Washington, D.C.: NCQA.

———. 2002. *State of Health Care Quality Report.* Washington, D.C.: NCQA.

National Conference of State Legislatures. "Influenza Vaccine Rates Among People Age 65 and Older." *Imunization Project.* Washington, D.C.

National Heart Lung and Blood Institute (NHLBI). 1998. "The NHLBI Clinical Guidelines." Online. Available at www.nhlbi.nih/.gov/guileines/obesity/e.textbk/index/htm [accessed Aug. 26, 2002].

National Institutes of Health. 2002. State-of-the-Science Conference Statement. *State-of-the-Science Conference on Symptom Management in Cancer: Pain, Depression, and Fatigue.* National Institutes of Health

Newacheck, P. W., M. A. McManus, and H. B. Fox. 1991. Prevalence and impact of chronic illness among adolescents. *Am J Dis Child* 145 (12):1367-73.

Newacheck, P. W., B. Strickland, J. P. Shonkoff, J. M. Perrin, M. McPherson, M. McManus, C. Lauver, H. Fox, and P. Arango. 1998. An epidemiologic profile of children with special health care needs. *Pediatrics* 102 (1 Pt 1):117-23.

Newacheck, P. W., and W. R. Taylor. 1992. Childhood chronic illness: Prevalence, severity, and impact. *Am J Public Health* 82 (3):364-71.

NHLBI USPHS. 1997. *Expert Panel Report 2. Guidelines for the Diagnosis and Management of Asthma.* Bethesda, MD: National Institutes of Health.

Ni, H., D. J. Nauman, and R. E. Hershberger. 1998. Managed care and outcomes of hospitalization among elderly patients with congestive heart failure. *Arch Intern Med* 158 (11):1231-6.

NIH Consensus Statement. 1996. Cervical cancer. 14 (1):1-38.

Nolan, T., I. Zvagulis, and B. Pless. 1987. Controlled trial of social work in childhood chronic illness. *Lancet* 2 (8556):411-5.

Norman, D. C. 2002. Management of antibiotic-resistant bacteria. *J Am Geriatr Soc* 50 (7 Suppl):S242-6.

Norris, S. L., M. M. Engelgau, and K. M. Narayan. 2001. Effectiveness of self-management training in type 2 diabetes: A systematic review of randomized controlled trials. *Diabetes Care* 24 (3):561-87.

Nyquist, A. C., R. Gonzales, J. F. Steiner, and M. A. Sande. 1998. Antibiotic prescribing for children with colds, upper respiratory tract infections, and bronchitis. *JAMA* 279 (11):875-7.

O'Connor, G. T., H. B. Quinton, N. D. Traven, L. D. Ramunno, T. A. Dodds, T. A. Marciniak, and J. E. Wennberg. 1999 . Geographic variation in the treatment of acute myocardial infarction: The Cooperative Cardiovascular Project. *JAMA* 281 (7):627-33.

Olivarius, N. F., H. Beck-Nielsen, A. H. Andreasen, M. Horder, and P. A. Pedersen. 2001. Randomised controlled trial of structured personal care of type 2 diabetes mellitus. *BMJ* 323 (7319):970-5.

Oliveria, S. A., P. Lapuerta, B. D. McCarthy, G. J. L'Italien, D. R. Berlowitz, and S. M. Asch. 2002. Physician-related barriers to the effective management of uncontrolled hypertension. *Arch Intern Med* 162 (4):413-20.

Ornish, D., L. W. Scherwitz, J. H. Billings, S. E. Brown, K. L. Gould, T. A. Merritt, S. Sparler, W. T. Armstrong, T. A. Ports, R. L. Kirkeide, C. Hogeboom, and R. J. Brand. 1998. Intensive lifestyle changes for reversal of coronary heart disease. *JAMA* 280 (23):2001-7.

Ossip-Klein, D. J., T. A. Pearson, S. McIntosh, and C. T. Orleans. 1999. Smoking is a geriatric health issue. *Nicotine Tob Res* 1 (4):299-300.

Partnership for Prevention. 1999. *Why Invest in Disease Prevention? It's a Good Business Decision. And It's Good for American Business.*

———. 2002. *Prevention Priorities: A Health Plan's Guide to the Highest Value Preventive Health Services.*

Partnership for Solutions, The Johns Hopkins University. 2001. "Partnership for Solutions: A National Program of The Robert Wood Johnson Foundation." Online. Available at http://www.partnershipforsolutions.org/statistics/prevalence.htm [accessed Dec. 12, 2002].

Perez-Stable, E. J., and E. Fuentes-Afflick. 1998. Role of clinicians in cigarette smoking prevention. *West J Med* 169 (1):23-9.

Perz, J. F., A. S. Craig, C. S. Coffey, D. M. Jorgensen, E. Mitchel, S. Hall, W. Schaffner, and M. R. Griffin. 2002. Changes in antibiotic prescribing for children after a community-wide campaign. *JAMA* 287 (23):3103-9.

Petersen, L. A., S. M. Wright, E. D. Peterson, and J. Daley. 2002. Impact of race on cardiac care and outcomes in veterans with acute myocardial infarction. *Med Care* 40 (1.Supp):86-96.

Pfizer. 1998. "Promoting Health Literacy: A Call to Action." Online. Available at http://www.pfizerhealthliteracy.com [accessed July 11, 2002].

Phillips, D. M. 2000. JCAHO pain management standards are unveiled. Joint Commission on Accreditation of Healthcare Organizations. *JAMA* 284 (4):428-9.

Phillips, D. P., N. Christenfeld, and L. M. Glynn. 1998. Increase in US medication-error deaths between 1983 and 1993. *Lancet* 351 (9103):643-4.

Phillips, J., S. Beam, A. Brinker, C. Holquist, P. Honig, L. Y. Lee, and C. Pamer. 2001. Retrospective analysis of mortalities associated with medication errors. *Am J Health Syst Pharm* 58 (19):1835-41.

Pignone, M., C. Phillips, and C. Mulrow. 2000. Use of lipid lowering drugs for primary prevention of coronary heart disease: Meta-analysis of randomised trials. *BMJ* 321 (7267):983-6.

Pignone, M., S. Saha, T. Hoerger, and J. Mandelblatt. 2002. Cost-effectiveness analyses of colorectal cancer screening: A systematic review for the U.S. Preventive Services Task Force. *Ann Intern Med* 137 (2):96-104.

Pilote, L., R. M. Califf, S. Sapp, D. P. Miller, D. B. Mark, W. D. Weaver, J. M. Gore, P. W. Armstrong, E. M. Ohman, and E. J. Topol. 1995. Regional variation across the United States in the management of acute myocardial infarction. GUSTO-1 Investigators. Global Utilization of Streptokinase and Tissue Plasminogen Activator for Occluded Coronary Arteries. *N Engl J Med* 333 (9):565-72.

Pincus, H. A., T. L. Tanielian, S. C. Marcus, M. Olfson, D. A. Zarin, J. Thompson, and J. Magno Zito. 1998. Prescribing trends in psychotropic medications: Primary care, psychiatry, and other medical specialties. *JAMA* 279 (7):526-31.

Pless, I. B. and M. E. Wadsworth. 1988. The unresolved question: Long-term psychological sequelae of chronic illness in childhood. In: R. E.K. Stein ed. *Caring for Children with Chronic Illness: Issues and Strategies.* New York, NY: Springer Publishing Company.

Post-stroke Rehabilitation Panel, GE Gresham Chair. 1995. *Post-stroke Rehabilitation.* Rockville, MD: Agency for Health Care Policy and Research.

Prevention Program Reduces Incidences of Pressure Ulcers by Up to 87%. 2002. *Dermatol Nurs* 14 (4):286.

Psaty, B. M., N. L. Smith, D. S. Siscovick, T. D. Koepsell, N. S. Weiss, S. R. Heckbert, R. N. Lemaitre, E. H. Wagner, and C. D. Furberg. 1997. Health outcomes associated with antihypertensive therapies used as first-line agents. A systematic review and meta-analysis. *JAMA* 277 (9):739-45.

Rathore, S. S., J. D. McGreevey 3rd, K. A. Schulman, and D. Atkins. 2000. Mandated coverage for cancer-screening services: Whose guidelines do states follow? *Am J Prev Med* 19 (2):71-8.

Renders, C. M., G. D. Valk, S. J. Griffin, E. H. Wagner, J. T. Eijk Van, and W. J. Assendelft. 2001. Interventions to improve the management of diabetes in primary care, outpatient, and community settings: A systematic review. *Diabetes Care* 24 (10):1821-33.

Rennels, M. B., and H. C. Meissner. 2002. Technical report: Reduction of the influenza burden in children. *Pediatrics* 110 (6):e80.

Reogowski J. 1998. Cost-effectiveness of care for very low birth weight infants. *Pediatrics* (102):35-43.

Rich, M. W. 1997. Epidemiology, pathophysiology, and etiology of congestive heart failure in older adults. *J Am Geriatr Soc* 45 (8):968-74.

———. 1999. Heart failure disease management: a critical review. *J Card Fail* 5 (1):64-75.

Richards, C., T. G. Emori, J. Edwards, S. Fridkin, J. Tolson, and R. Gaynes. 2001. Characteristics of hospital and infection control professionals participating in the National Nosocomial Infections Surveillance System 1999. *Am J Infect Control* 29 (6):400-403.

Ries, L. A., M. P. Eisner, and C. L. Kosary. 2002. *SEER Cancer Statistics Review, 1973-1999.* Bethesda, MD: National Cancer Institute, 2002.

Rimer, B. K., C. T. Orleans, M. K. Keintz, S. Cristinzio, and L. Fleisher. 1990. The older smoker. Status, challenges and opportunities for intervention. *Chest* 97 (3):547-53.

Rodewald, L. E., P. G. Szilagyi, S. G. Humiston, R. Barth, R. Kraus, and R. F. Raubertas. 1999. A randomized study of tracking with outreach and provider prompting to improve immunization coverage and primary care. *Pediatrics* 103 (1):31-8.

Rogowski, J. 1998. Cost-effectiveness of care for very low birth weight infants. *Pediatrics* 102 (1 Pt 1):35-43.

Rosenberg, C. H., and G. M. Popelka. 2000. Post-stroke rehabilitation. A review of the guidelines for patient management. *Geriatrics* 55 (9):75-81; quiz 82.

Rosenheck, R. A., and D. Dennis. 2001. Time-limited assertive community treatment for homeless persons with severe mental illness. *Arch Gen Psychiatry* 58 (11):1073-80.

Roth, E. J., A. W. Heinemann, L. L. Lovell, R. L. Harvey, J. R. McGuire, and S. Diaz. 1998. Impairment and disability: Their relation during stroke rehabilitation. *Arch Phys Med Rehabil* 79 (3):329-35.

Roth, K., J. Lynn, Z. Zhong, M. Borum, and N. V. Dawson. 2000. Dying with end stage liver disease with cirrhosis: Insights from SUPPORT. Study to Understand Prognoses and Preferences for Outcomes and Risks of Treatment. *J Am Geriatr Soc* 48 (5 Suppl):S122-30.

Saaddine, J. B., M. M. Engelgau, G. L. Beckles, E. W. Gregg, T. J. Thompson, and K. M. Narayan. 2002. A diabetes report card for the United States: Quality of care in the 1990s. *Ann Intern Med* 136 (8):565-74.

Sacchetti, A., M. Gerardi, R. Barkin, J. Santamaria, R. Cantor, J. Weinberg, and M. Gausche. 1996. Emergency data set for children with special needs. *Ann Emerg Med* 28 (3):324-7.

Sadur, C. N., N. Moline, M. Costa, D. Michalik, D. Mendlowitz, S. Roller, R. Watson, B. E. Swain, J. V. Selby, and W. C. Javorski. 1999. Diabetes management in a health maintenance organization. Efficacy of care management using cluster visits. *Diabetes Care* 22 (12):2011-7.

Samsa, G. P., D. B. Matchar, L. B. Goldstein, A. J. Bonito, L. J. Lux, D. M. Witter, and J. Bian. 2000. Quality of anticoagulation management among patients with atrial fibrillation: Results of a review of medical records from 2 communities. *Arch Intern Med* 160 (7):967-73.

Saslow, D., C. D. Runowicz, D. Solomon, A.-B. Moscicki, R. A. Smith, H. J. Eyre, and C. Cohen. 2002. American Cancer Society Guideline for the Early Detection of Cervical Neoplasia and Cancer. *CA Cancer J Clin* 52 (6):342-62.

Sawaya, G. F., and D. A. Grimes. 1999. New technologies in cervical cytology screening: A word of caution. *Obstet Gynecol* 94 (2):307-10.

Schappert, S. M. 1997. Ambulatory care visits of physician offices, hospital outpatient departments, and emergency departments: United States, 1995. *Vital Health Stat 13* (129):1-38.

Schillinger, D., K. Grumbach, J. Piette, F. Wang, D. Osmond, C. Daher, J. Palacios, G. D. Sullivan, and A. B. Bindman. 2002. Association of health literacy with diabetes outcomes. *JAMA* 288 (4):475-82.

Schlesinger, M., R. Dorwart, C. Hoover, and S. Epstein. 1997. The determinants of dumping: A national study of economically motivated transfers involving mental health care. *Health Serv Res* 32 (5):561-90.

Schneider, E. C., A. M. Zaslavsky, and A. M. Epstein. 2002. Racial disparities in the quality of care for enrollees in medicare managed care. *JAMA* 287 (10):1288-94.

Schoenbaum, M., J. Unutzer, C. Sherbourne, N. Duan, L. V. Rubenstein, J. Miranda, L. S. Meredith, M. F. Carney, and K. Wells. 2001. Cost-effectiveness of practice-initiated quality improvement for depression: Results of a randomized controlled trial. *JAMA* 286 (11):1325-30 .

Schulberg, H. C., W. Katon, G. E. Simon, and A. J. Rush. 1998. Treating major depression in primary care practice: An update of the Agency for Health Care Policy and Research Practice Guidelines. *Arch Gen Psychiatry* 55 (12):1121-7.

Schulman, K. A., J. A. Berlin, W. Harless, J. F. Kerner, S. Sistrunk, B. J. Gersh, R. Dube, C. K. Taleghani, J. E. Burke, S. Williams, J. M. Eisenberg, and J. J. Escarce. 1999. The effect of race and sex on physicians' recommendations for cardiac catheterization. *N Engl J Med* 340 (8):618-26.

Schwartz, C. E., H. B. Wheeler, B. Hammes, N. Basque, J. Edmunds, G. Reed, Y. Ma, L. Li, P. Tabloski, and J. Yanko. 2002. Early intervention in planning end-of-life care with ambulatory geriatric patients: Results of a pilot trial. *Arch Intern Med* 162 (14):1611-8.

Scott, J. G., D. Cohen, B. DiCicco-Bloom, A. J. Orzano, C. R. Jaen, and B. F. Crabtree. 2001. Antibiotic use in acute respiratory infections and the ways patients pressure physicians for a prescription. *J Fam Pract* 50 (10):853-8.

Seeff, L. C., J. A. Shapiro, and M. R. Nadel. 2002. Are we doing enough to screen for colorectal cancer? Findings from the 1999 Behavioral Risk Factor Surveillance System. *J Fam Pract* 51 (9):761-6.

Senate report number 102-397.

Serdula, M. K., A. H. Mokdad, D. F. Williamson, D. A. Galuska, J. M. Mendlein, and G. W. Heath. 1999. Prevalence of attempting weight loss and strategies for controlling weight. *JAMA* 282 (14):1353-8.

Sheikh, K., and C. Bullock. 2001. Urban-rural differences in the quality of care for medicare patients with acute myocardial infarction. *Arch Intern Med* 161 (5):737-43.

Shipp, M., M. S. Croughan-Minihane, D. B. Petitti, and A. E. Washington. 1992. Estimation of the break-even point for smoking cessation programs in pregnancy. *Am J Public Health* 82 (3):383-90.

Shortell, S. M., R. R. Gillies, and D. A. Anderson. 2000. *Remaking Health Care in America.* 2nd edition. San Francisco, CA: Jossey-Bass.

Silber, J. H., S. P. Gleeson, and H. Zhao. 1999. The influence of chronic disease on resource utilization in common acute pediatric conditions. Financial concerns for children's hospitals. *Arch Pediatr Adolesc Med* 153 (2):169-79.

Simon, G. E., D. Goldberg, B. G. Tiemens, and T. B. Ustun. 1999. Outcomes of recognized and unrecognized depression in an international primary care study. *Gen Hosp Psychiatry* 21 (2):97-105.

Simon, G. E., M. VonKorff, C. Rutter, and E. Wagner. 2000. Randomised trial of monitoring, feedback, and management of care by telephone to improve treatment of depression in primary care. *BMJ* 320 (7234):550-4.

Sloan, P. A., B. L. Vanderveer, J. S. Snapp, M. Johnson, and D. A. Sloan. 1999. Cancer pain assessment and management recommendations by hospice nurses. University of Kentucky, Lexington, KY. *J Pain Symptom Manage* 18 (2):103-10.

Solberg, L. I., T. E. Kottke, S. A. Conn, M. L. Brekke, C. A. Calomeni, and K. S. Conboy. 1997. Delivering clinical preventive services is a systems problem. *Ann Behav Med* 19 (3):271-8.

Sperl-Hillen, J., P. J. O'Connor, R. R. Carlson, T. B. Lawson, C. Halstenson, T. Crowson, and J. Wuorenma. 2000. Improving diabetes care in a large health care system: an enhanced primary care approach. *Jt Comm J Qual Improv* 26 (11):615-22.

Spore, D. L., V. Mor, P. Larrat, C. Hawes, and J. Hiris. 1997. Inappropriate drug prescriptions for elderly residents of board and care facilities. *Am J Public Health* 87 (3):404-9.

Squires, S. Dec. 13, 2001. Surgeon General Outlines National Plan on Obesity. *The Washington Post.*

St Lawrence, J. S., D. E. Montano, D. Kasprzyk, W. R. Phillips, K. Armstrong, and J. S. Leichliter. 2002. STD screening, testing, case reporting, and clinical and partner notification practices: A national survey of US physicians. *Am J Public Health* 92 (11):1784-8.

Standards for the diagnosis and care of patients with chronic obstructive pulmonary disease. American Thoracic Society. 1995. *Am J Respir Crit Care Med* 152 (5 Pt 2):S77-121.

STAR*D Program. "Sequenced treatment alternatives to relieve depression." Online. Available at http://www.edc.gsph.pitt.edu/stard [accessed July, 2002].

Stein, R. 1983. A home care program for children with chronic illness. *Child Health Care* 12 (2):90-2.

Stone, E. G., S. C. Morton, M. E. Hulscher, M. A. Maglione, E. A. Roth, J. M. Grimshaw, B. S. Mittman, L. V. Rubenstein, L. Z. Rubenstein , and P. G. Shekelle. 2002. Interventions that increase use of adult immunization and cancer screening services: A meta-analysis. *Ann Intern Med* 136 (9):641-51.

Strauss, R. S., and H. A. Pollack. 2001. Epidemic increase in childhood overweight, 1986-1998. *JAMA* 286 (22):2845-8.

Stuck, A. E., M. H. Beers, A. Steiner, H. U. Aronow, L. Z. Rubenstein, and J. C. Beck. 1994. Inappropriate medication use in community-residing older persons. *Arch Intern Med* 154 (19):2195-200.

Sturm, R. 1999. Tracking changes in behavioral health services: How have carve-outs changed care? *J Behav Health Serv Res* 26 (4):360-71.

Sturm, R. 2002. The effects of obesity, smoking, and drinking on medical problems and costs. Obesity outranks both smoking and drinking in its deleterious effects on health and health costs. *Health Aff (Millwood)* 21 (2):245-53.

Tamminga, C. A. 1997. Gender and schizophrenia. *J Clin Psychiatry* 58Suppl 15:33-7.

Taylor, D. H. Jr, V. Hasselblad, S. J. Henley, M. J. Thun, and F. A. Sloan. 2002. Benefits of smoking cessation for longevity. *Am J Public Health* 92 (6):990-6.

Testa, M. A., and D. C. Simonson. 1998. Health economic benefits and quality of life during improved glycemic control in patients with type 2 diabetes mellitus: A randomized, controlled, double-blind trial. *JAMA* 280 (17):1490-6.

The Commonwealth Fund. 2002. *Quality of Health Care in the United States: A Chartbook.*

The National Coalition on Health Care and the Institute for Healthcare Improvement. 2002. *Curing the System: Stories of Change in Chronic Illness Care.*The National Coalition on Health Care and the Institute for Healthcare Improvement.

The Robert Wood Johnson Foundation. 2001. *Substance Abuse: The Nation's Number One Health Problem.* Princeton, NJ: Robert Wood Johnson Foundation.

————. 2002. *National Partnership to Help Pregnant Smokers Quit: Action Plan.* Princeton, NJ: Robert Wood Johnson Foundation.

The sixth report of the Joint National Committee on prevention, detection, evaluation, and treatment of high blood pressure. 1997. *Arch Intern Med* 157 (21):2413-46.

Thompson, R. S. 1996. What have HMOs learned about clinical prevention services? An examination of the experience at Group Health Cooperative of Puget Sound. *Milbank Q* 74 (4):469-509.

Thorndike, A. N., N. A. Rigotti, R. S. Stafford, and D. E. Singer. 1998. National patterns in the treatment of smokers by physicians. *JAMA* 279 (8):604-8.

Thornley, B., C. E. Adams, and G. Awad. 2000. Chlorpromazine versus placebo for schizophrenia. *Cochrane Database Syst Rev* (2):CD000284.

Tinetti, M. E., and C. S. Williams. 1998. The effect of falls and fall injuries on functioning in community- dwelling older persons. *J Gerontol A Biol Sci Med Sci* 53 (2):M112-9.

Tomar, S. L., C. G. Husten, and M. W. Manley . 1996. Do dentists and physicians advise tobacco users to quit? *J Am Dent Assoc* 127 (2):259-65.

Trepka, M. J., E. A. Belongia, P. H. Chyou, J. P. Davis, and B. Schwartz. 2001. The effect of a community intervention trial on parental knowledge and awareness of antibiotic resistance and appropriate antibiotic use in children. *Pediatrics* 107 (1):E6.

United States Department of Health and Human Services. 1990. *The Health Benefits of Smoking Cessation: A Report of the Surgeon General.* Vol. Rockland, MD: U.S. Govenment Printing Office.

————. 1998. "National Vital Statistics Reports." Washington, D.C.: Department of Health and Human Services.

————. 2000. *Healthy People 2010: Understanding and Improving Health.* 2nd edition. Washington, D.C.: U.S. Government Printing Office.

————. 2001a. *The Surgeon General's Call to Action to Prevent and Decrease Overweight and Obesity.* Vol. Rockville, MD: U.S. Department of Health and Human Services, Public Health Services, Office of the Surgeon General.

————. 2001b. *Women and Smoking : A Report of the Surgeon General.* Vol. Rockland, MD: U.S. Govenment Printing Office.

————. 2002. "National Vital Statistics Reports." Washington, D.C.: CDC—Centers for Disease Control and Prevention.

United States General Accounting Office. 2000. *Medicaid Managed Care: Challenges in Implementing Safeguards for Children with Special Needs.* Washington, D.C.: U.S. Goverment Printing Office.

United States Preventive Services Task Force. 1996. *Guide to Clinical Preventive Services.* Baltimore, MD: Williams and Wilkins.

United States Preventive Services Task Force. 2002a. Behavioral counseling in primary care to promote a physical activity: Recommendation and rationale. *Ann Intern Med* 137:205-8.

United States Preventive Services Task Force. 2002b. "Recommendations and Rationale: Screening for Colorectal Cancer." Online. Available at http://www.ahrq.gov/ clinic/3rduspstf/colorectal/colorr.htm [accessed Nov. 20, 2002b].

United States Preventive Services Task Force. 2003. Behavioral counseling primary care to promote a healthy diet. Recommendation and rationale. *Am J Prev Med* 24(1):93-100

United States Public Health Service. 1999. Office of the Surgeon General Mental Health: A Report of the Surgeon General. pp 244-68.

van der Lee, J. H., R. C. Wagenaar, G. J. Lankhorst, T. W. Vogelaar, W. L. Deville, and L. M. Bouter. 1999. Forced use of the upper extremity in chronic stroke patients: Results from a single-blind randomized clinical trial. *Stroke* 30 (11):2369-75.

Vasan, R. S., A. Beiser, S. Seshadri, M. G. Larson, W. B. Kannel, R. B. D'Agostino, and D. Levy. 2002. Residual lifetime risk for developing hypertension in middle-aged women and men: The Framingham Heart Study. *JAMA* 287 (8):1003-10.

Verschuren, W. M., D. R. Jacobs, B. P. Bloemberg, D. Kromhout, A. Menotti, C. Aravanis, H. Blackburn, R. Buzina, A. S. Dontas, and F. Fidanza. 1995. Serum total cholesterol and long-term coronary heart disease mortality in different cultures. Twenty-five-year follow-up of the seven countries study. *JAMA* 274 (2):131-6.

Vintzileos, A. M., C. V. Ananth, J. C. Smulian, W. E. Scorza, and R. A. Knuppel. 2002. The impact of prenatal care on neonatal deaths in the presence and absence of antenatal high-risk conditions. *Am J Obstet Gynecol* 186 (5):1011-6.

Vishnu-Priya, S., H. Izurieta, C. Bridges, E. Bolyard, D. Johnson, and M. Hoyt. 2000. Prevention and Control of Vaccine-Preventable Diseases in Long-Term Care Facilities. *Journal of American Medical Directors Association* :S2-S37.

Viskin, S., and H. V. Barron. 1996. Beta blockers prevent cardiac death following a myocardial infarction: So why are so many infarct survivors discharged without beta blockers? *Am J Cardiol* 78 (7):821-2.

Von Korff, M., J. Gruman, J. Schaefer, S. J. Curry, and E. H. Wagner. 1997. Collaborative management of chronic illness. *Ann Intern Med* 127 (12):1097-102.

Von Korff, M., G. Nestadt, A. Romanoski, J. Anthony, W. Eaton, A. Merchant, R. Chahal, M. Kramer, M. Folstein, and E. Gruenberg. 1985. Prevalence of treated and untreated DSM-III schizophrenia. Results of a two-stage community survey. *J Nerv Ment Dis* 173 (10):577-81.

Wadden, T. A., and G. D. Foster. 2000. Behavioral treatment of obesity. *Med Clin North Am* 84 (2):441-61, vii.

Wagner, E. H., S. J. Curry, L. Grothaus, K. W. Saunders, and C. M. McBride. 1995. The impact of smoking and quitting on health care use. *Arch Intern Med* 155 (16):1789-95.

Wagner, E. H., B. T. Austin, and M. Von Korff. 1996. Organizing care for patients with chronic illness. *Milbank Q* 74 (4):511-44.

Wagner, E. H., R. E. Glasgow, C. Davis, A. E. Bonomi, L. Provost, D. McCulloch, P. Carver, and C. Sixta. 2001a. Quality improvement in chronic illness care: A collaborative approach. *Jt Comm J Qual Improv* 27 (2):63-80.

Wagner, E. H., N. Sandhu, K. M. Newton, D. K. McCulloch, S. D. Ramsey, and L. C. Grothaus. 2001b. Effect of improved glycemic control on health care costs and utilization. *JAMA* 285 (2):182-9.

Wagner, E. H., B. T. Austin, C. Davis, M. Hindmarsh, J. Schaefer, and A. Bonomi. 2001c. Improving chronic illness care: Translating evidence into action. *Health Aff (Millwood)* 20 (6):64-78.

Wahlbeck, K., M. Cheine, and M. A. Essali. 2000. Clozapine versus typical neuroleptic medication for schizophrenia. *Cochrane Database Syst Rev* (2):CD000059.

Wallander, J. L., J. W. Varni, L. Babani, H. T. Banis, and K. T. Wilcox. 1988. Children with chronic physical disorders: Maternal reports of their psychological adjustment. *J Pediatr Psychol* 13 (2):197-212.

Wallander, J. L., J. W. Varni, L. Babani, C. B. DeHaan, K. T. Wilcox, and H. T. Banis. 1989. The social environment and the adaptation of mothers of physically handicapped children. *J Pediatr Psychol* 14 (3):371-87.

Walston, J., and L. P. Fried. 1999. Frailty and the older man. *Med Clin North Am* 83 (5):1173-94.

Wang, P. S., P. Berglund, and R. C. Kessler. 2000. Recent care of common mental disorders in the United States: Prevalence and conformance with evidence-based recommendations. *J Gen Intern Med* 15 (5):284-92.

Wang, P. S., O. Demler, and R. C. Kessler. 2002. Adequacy of treatment for serious mental illness in the United States. *Am J Public Health* 92 (1):92-8.

Weaver, W. D., R. J. Simes, A. Betriu, C. L. Grines, F. Zijlstra, E. Garcia, L. Grinfeld, R. J. Gibbons, E. E. Ribeiro, M. A. DeWood, and F. Ribichini. 1997. Comparison of primary coronary angioplasty and intravenous thrombolytic therapy for acute myocardial infarction: A quantitative review. *JAMA* 278 (23):2093-8.

Weiland, S. K., I. B. Pless, and K. J. Roghmann. 1992. Chronic illness and mental health problems in pediatric practice: Results from a survey of primary care providers. *Pediatrics* 89 (3):445-9.

Weinstein, R. A. 1998. Nosocomial infection update. *Emerg Infect Dis* 4 (3):416-20.

Weiss, K. B., and S. D. Sullivan. 2001. The health economics of asthma and rhinitis. I. Assessing the economic impact. *J Allergy Clin Immunol* 107 (1):3-8.

Weiss, K. B., S. D. Sullivan, and C. S. Lyttle. 2000. Trends in the cost of illness for asthma in the United States, 1985-1994. *J Allergy Clin Immunol* 106 (3):493-9.

Wells, K.B. 2002a. *Mental Disorders and Candidate Quality Improvement Conditions.* Presented at May 9-10, 2002 Priority Areas for Quality Improvement Meeting.

Wells, K.B. 2002b. The story and findings of Partners in Care. From Jackson-Triche M, Wells KB, Minnium K. Beating Depression: The Journey to Hope. New York: McGraw Hill.

Wells, K. B., C. Sherbourne, M. Schoenbaum, N. Duan, L. Meredith, J. Unutzer, J. Miranda, M. F. Carney, and L. V. Rubenstein. 2000. Impact of disseminating quality improvement programs for depression in managed primary care: A randomized controlled trial. *JAMA* 283 (2):212-20.

Wells, K. B., A. Stewart, R. D. Hays, M. A. Burnam, W. Rogers, M. Daniels, S. Berry, S. Greenfield, and J. Ware. 1989. The functioning and well-being of depressed patients. Results from the Medical Outcomes Study. *JAMA* 262 (7):914-9.

Wenzel, R. P., and M. B. Edmond. 2001. The impact of hospital-acquired bloodstream infections. *Emerg Infect Dis* 7 (2):174-7.

Whelton, P. K., J. He, L. J. Appel, J. A. Cutler, S. Havas, T. A. Kotchen, E. J. Roccella, R. Stout, C. Vallbona, M. C. Winston, and J. Karimbakas. 2002. Primary prevention of hypertension: Clinical and public health advisory from the national high blood pressure education program. *JAMA* 288 (15):1882-8.

Whitney, C. G., M. M. Farley, J. Hadler, L. H. Harrison, C. Lexau, A. Reingold, L. Lefkowitz, P. R. Cieslak, M. Cetron, E. R. Zell, J. H. Jorgensen, and A. Schuchat. 2000. Increasing prevalence of multidrug-resistant streptococcus pneumoniae in the United States. *N Engl J Med* 343 (26):1917-24.

Willcox, S. M., D. U. Himmelstein, and S. Woolhandler. 1994. Inappropriate drug prescribing for the community-dwelling elderly. *JAMA* 272 (4):292-6.

Wisborg, K., T. B. Henriksen, C. Obel, E. Skajaa, and J. R. Ostergaard. 1999. Smoking during pregnancy and hospitalization of the child. *Pediatrics* 104 (4):e46.

World Health Organization. 1996. With a guide to opioid availability. *Cancer Pain Relief.* 2nd edition. Geneva: World Health Organization.

————. 2000. "Global Burden of Disease 2000 Version 1 Estimates." Online. Available at http://www3.who.int/whosis/menu [accessed May 29, 2002].

Yanovski, S. Z., and J. A. Yanovski. 2002. Obesity. *N Engl J Med* 346 (8):591-602.

Young, A. S., R. Klap, C. D. Sherbourne, and K. B. Wells. 2001. The quality of care for depressive and anxiety disorders in the United States. *Arch Gen Psychiatry* 58 (1):55-61.

Yusuf, S., R. Peto, J. Lewis, R. Collins, and P. Sleight. 1985. Beta blockade during and after myocardial infarction: An overview of the randomized trials. *Prog Cardiovasc Dis* 27 (5):335-71.

Zech, D. F., S. Grond, J. Lynch, D. Hertel, and K. A. Lehmann. 1995. Validation of World Health Organization Guidelines for cancer pain relief: A 10-year prospective study. *Pain* 63 (1):65-76.

Zeiger, R. S., S. Heller, M. H. Mellon, J. Wald, R. Falkoff, and M. Schatz. 1991. Facilitated referral to asthma specialist reduces relapses in asthma emergency room visits. *J Allergy Clin Immunol* 87 (6):1160-8.

Zhan, C., J. Sangl, A. S. Bierman, M. R. Miller, B. Friedman, S. W. Wickizer, and G. S. Meyer. 2001. Potentially inappropriate medication use in the community-dwelling elderly: Findings from the 1996 Medical Expenditure Panel Survey. *JAMA* 286 (22):2823-9.

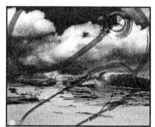

Chapter Four
Process for Identifying Priority Areas

Guiding Principles

The initial set of priority areas was chosen to guide the nation in taking the first steps toward a systematic redesign of the health care system. As discussed in Chapter 2, the committee focused on areas that have a high impact; are most amenable to improvement; and are broadly inclusive in several respects, cutting across the entire life span, involving the continuum of care from disease prevention through the end of life, and affecting a range of demographic groups for which inequities in health care need to be redressed.

The committee developed its recommendations using an evidence-based approach, supplemented by the perspectives of experienced experts. It relied on quantitative data from national datasets to compare the burden of disease for specific conditions, evaluating such items as population-based estimates for prevalence and costs. The design of these measures allows for estimates of ranking and for rough comparisons across conditions. The committee synthesized available evidence from the literature and experience to judge the extent of improvability for each area through systems change.

The salient studies do not share common interventions or outcome measures and are often not reported in the published literature. Thus, the committee took both a quantitative and qualitative approach when assessing the potential for systems change, and employed data as well as the negotiated consensus of the group to decide whether a priority area under consideration met a threshold of confidence for improvability. The committee also considered the degree to which effective systems change in one area had the potential to diffuse to other areas in which improvements would be welcome. Making this determination required judgment as well, as there can be no historical evidence for the ability of improvement in one priority area to generate improvement in similar conditions or settings until systems changes have actually been implemented. Thus the committee turned to illuminating examples of systems transformation provided by workshop presenters and presented in the literature, and took into account the value of these experiences.

Recognizing that no priority-setting process is perfect, the committee believed it essential to make its process as transparent as possible, being clear and open about the bases for its decisions (Daniels, 2000; Daniels and Sabin, 1998). The committee also decided that the process it adopted would have to be dynamic, capable of evolving over time, and characterized by ongoing interaction among its various components. A feedback loop would be needed as well to allow for periodic revisiting and updating of the priority areas and continuous assessment of progress.

This chapter describes the process used by the committee to identify the priority areas in the brief period of time available for this study. Additionally, a revised process is recommended for the future determination of priority areas, based upon the committee's experience with its initial process.

Process use by the Committee

The process used by the committee, summarized in Figure 4-1, consists of the following steps:

1. Determine a framework for the priority areas.

2. Identify candidate priority areas.

3. Establish criteria for selecting the final priority areas.

4. Categorize candidate areas within the framework.

5. Apply criteria to screen the candidates.

6. Identify priority areas; reassess and approve.

Although the process appears to be linear in fashion, it is much more dynamic than a succession of orderly steps. The decisions required in the first three steps, for example, are all closely interrelated.

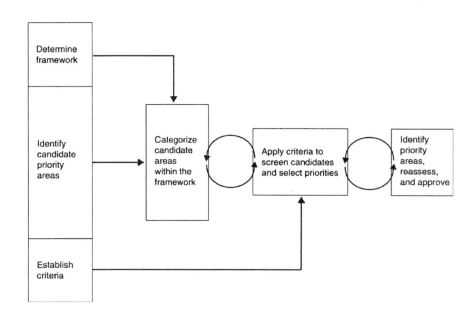

FIGURE 4-1 Process model used by the committee.

Determine Framework

The framework used by the committee is discussed in Chapter 1.

Identify Candidate Priority Areas

In developing an initial candidate list, the committee drew on a variety of sources. In addition to the collective knowledge and broad expertise of its members, the committee made use of feedback received from presenters and the public at a workshop held in May 2002 (see Chapter 1 for a brief description of the workshop and Appendix B for its agenda).

The committee also considered the work done by other groups in the area of the burden of chronic conditions/diseases. It reviewed datasets on the economic burden of chronic diseases compiled by the Medical Expenditure Panel Survey, (Cohen, 2001; Medical Expenditure Panel Survey, 2002) and the Centers for Disease Control and Prevention (CDC) (2000, 2002). In addition, although this study's focus was national, the committee considered statistics from the Global Burden of Disease Study (Michaud et al., 2001; Murray and Lopez, 1996). The committee also reviewed many of the Health Plan Employer Data and Information Set (HEDIS®) standardized performance measures currently used by the National Committee for Quality Assurance (NCQA) in its accreditation process (National Committee for Quality Assurance, 2002).

The committee then looked to the work of other groups that have established lists of targeted or priority conditions and areas to meet their specific needs. These groups included the Agency for Healthcare Research and Quality's (AHRQ) MEPS, the Veterans Administration's (VA) Quality Enhancement Research Initiative (QUERI), the Health Resources and Services Administration's (HRSA) Health Disparities Collaboratives, and the Centers for Medicare and Medicaid Services' (CMS) Quality Improvement Program (see Table 4-1 and Appendix C for more detail). To examine priorities pertaining to preventive services, the committee considered the work of Partnership for Prevention (see Table 4-2 and Appendix C). In addition, although the setting of research priorities was outside the purview of this committee, the criteria employed by the National Institutes of Health (NIH) for assessing health needs[1] proved helpful in balancing the criteria established for screening candidate priority areas (see Appendix C). After utilizing all of the above resources, the committee compiled a list of over 60 candidate priority areas.

Establish Criteria

The criteria used by the committee in selecting the priority areas are described in Chapter 2.

Categorize Candidate Areas Within the Framework

Once a pool of candidate areas had been established, the candidates were organized within the categories of the framework. For example, the committee placed diabetes under chronic care, tobacco dependence treatment under preventive care, pain control under palliative care, acute respiratory infection under acute care, and care coordination under cross-cutting systems interventions. At this point, it became evident to the committee that the framework was a useful organizing tool, but its categories were too rigid. Many of the initial candidates fell quite easily into more than one category. For example, stroke could be viewed as the start of a chronic condition or an acute episode. Cancer could fall under chronic conditions, or it could perhaps be more appropriately placed under preventative care, such as screening for colorectal cancer.

---

[1] Number of people with a disease, number of deaths caused by a disease, degree of disability caused by a disease, degree to which a disease shortens a normal productive lifetime, economic and social costs of a disease, and the need to respond rapidly to control the spread of a disease (National Institutes of Health (NIH), 1997)

Although appearing in more than one category was a type of triangulation, it also exposed a weakness of this classification scheme. Nonetheless, while remaining cognizant of this limitation, the committee proceeded to organize the first-cut list of candidates in this fashion to facilitate application of the process model. In later deliberations and in determination of the final list of priority areas, the committee shifted away from placing areas within these categories and instead used the categories as part of a test of inclusiveness across the spectrum of areas. The framework thus served as a useful screen at the end of the process to assess the balance of the portfolio.

Being mindful that the number of priority areas requested by AHRQ was approximately 15 but no more than 20, the committee at this point set preliminary targets for the final portfolio of areas from each category of the framework. Chronic conditions received the largest allocation of approximately 8 final candidates because they were seen as far-reaching in their ability to spark change. Each of the other four categories of the framework (preventive care, acute care, palliative care, and cross-cutting systems interventions) was assigned approximately 3 areas each. As noted earlier, the committee believed it important to include on the final list a few cross-cutting areas (as opposed to specific conditions) that could be broadly applied to improve health care quality, especially since it was not possible to select every condition worthy of improvement.

Apply Criteria to Screen Candidates

After identifying a list of candidate priority areas and categorizing them within the framework, the committee applied the impact, inclusiveness, and improvability criteria to each candidate, being particularly sensitive to the impact on disadvantaged populations. Two subgroups were formed to accomplish this task. One group examined the areas within the chronic, acute, and palliative care categories; the other analyzed those within the categories of preventive care and cross-cutting systems

interventions. To facilitate this step, a matrix was developed in which each priority candidate was cross-referenced against the criteria. The cells of the matrix were then filled in with supporting data and their source.

Identify Priority Areas

The subgroups discussed the extent to which each of the candidates met the criteria and ranked them accordingly. They then selected their top candidates for presentation to the full committee. The committee discussed each of the proposed candidates, continually comparing them against the criteria. During these deliberations, some areas were refined and narrowed, while others were broadened. The committee then approved a final list. Candidates not chosen were eliminated because they were relatively weak on the impact or inclusiveness criterion. Others did not meet the improvability criterion because of a lack of scientific evidence and clinical guidelines for effective interventions and valid and reliable measures; these represent important needs for future research. See Chapter 3 for the committee's recommended list of priority areas.

TABLE 4-1 Comparison of Priority Areas from Selected Sources

Condition	AHRQ/MEPS	VA/QUERI	HRSA/ Collaboratives	CMS/Quality Improvement Program
Diabetes	✓	✓	✓	✓
Congestive Heart Failure		✓	✓	✓
Ischemic Heart Disease	✓	✓		
Hypertension	✓		✓	
Acute Myocardial Infarction			✓	✓
Stroke	✓	✓		
Depression/Mental Health		✓	✓	
Asthma	✓		✓	
HIV/AIDS		✓	✓	
Breast Cancer			✓a	✓
Cervical Cancer			✓a	
Colon Cancer			✓a	
Arthritis	✓			
COPDb	✓			
Spinal Cord Injury		✓		
Post Operative Infections				✓
Pneumonia				✓
Infant Mortality			✓a	
Immunization			✓a	

a Expected future collaboratives.
b COPD = chronic obstructive pulmonary disease

SOURCES: AHRQ/MEPS–(Cohen, 2002; Medical Expenditure Panel Survey, 2002); VA/QUERI–(Demakis et al., 2000; Feussner et al., 2000; Kizer et al., 2000). HRSA/Collaboratives–(Health Disparities Collaboratives, 2002; Stevens, 2002) CMS/Quality Improvement Program–D. Schulke, The American Health Quality Association, personal communication.

TABLE 4-2   Partnership for Prevention Priority Areas

Type of Service	Services Delivered to Less Than 50% of Target Population
Counseling	Tobacco cessation for adults Alcohol and drug abstinence for adolescents Antitobacco message or advice to quit to adolescents Problem drinking for adults
Screening	Vision impairment among adults aged 65+ Colorectal cancer (fecal occult blood test and/or sigmoidoscopy) among all persons aged 50+ Chlamydia among women aged 15-24 Problem drinking
Vaccine	Adults > age 65 for pneumococcal disease

SOURCE: Adapted from (Partnership for Prevention, 2002).

Recommended Process for Determining Priority Areas

As noted, several valuable lessons were learned as the committee was applying the above process. This section presents the committee's recommendations for further refinements to the process based upon these insights and assuming a longer time period for deliberations.

Since the committee's task was over once it had identified the priority areas, its process did not include implementation and outcome assessment. The recommended model includes these critical follow-up components: implementing strategies for improving care in the priority areas, evaluating their outcomes, and reviewing/updating the list of priority areas. Figure 4-2 presents the committee's recommended process for determining priority areas for a full and complete review. In this model, public input is solicited from multiple sources at all stages. The recommended process can be summarized as follows:

1. Determine a framework for the priority areas.

2. Identify candidate areas.

3. Establish criteria for selecting the final priority areas.

4. Categorize candidate areas within the framework.

5. Apply impact and inclusiveness criteria to the candidates.

6. Apply criteria of improvability and inclusiveness to the preliminary set of areas obtained in step 5.

7. Identify priority areas; reassess and approve.

8. Implement strategies for improving care in the priority areas, measure the impact of implementation, and review/update the list of areas.

Each step in this recommended process is discussed below.

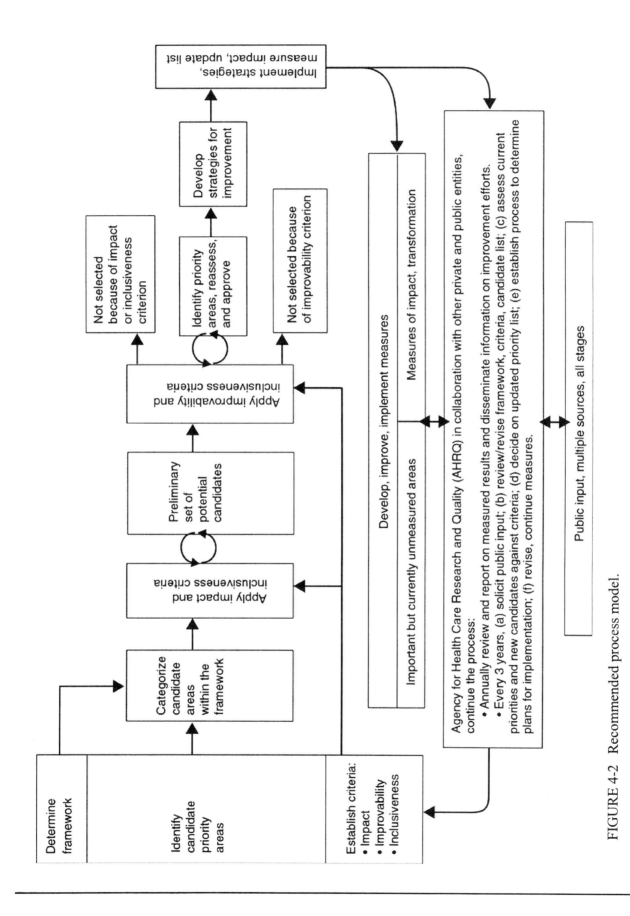

FIGURE 4-2 Recommended process model.

Determine Framework

As noted, the initial framework used by the committee was advantageous for some purposes, such as the initial identification of candidates, but it was also found to be overly constricting. Given this limitation, future priority-setting processes will need to strike a balance between the need for categorization and the desire to capture the more dynamic and complex processes taking place for patients in the real world.

Identify Candidate Priority Areas

To identify potential candidates, an extensive review of relevant data should be conducted, as well as a thorough synthesis of similar work done by other groups. Input from the public should be aggressively solicited. In addition, future processes will need to examine:

- Candidates that may become worthy of inclusion because issues associated with an area emerge, or measures are improved to allow more specificity about issues previously not measured, such as functional capacity.

- Outcomes of efforts to improve quality in the initial priority areas to determine whether to retain or replace them on the list.

- Candidates set aside in the past because of limits on the total number of priority areas, as well as improvability or measurement issues, to see whether changes have occurred that warrant their inclusion.

Establish Criteria

The criteria used by the committee are described in Chapter 2.

Categorize Candidate Areas Within the Framework

If a framework is used, the next step is to place the candidate areas into its categories.

Chapter 1 details the initial framework adopted by the committee.

Apply Impact and Inclusiveness Criteria

Next, the impact and inclusiveness criteria should be applied to the initial pool of candidates using available data and public input. At this stage, individual areas should be ranked in terms of their clinical burden. A variety of data sources should be compared to ensure balance and inclusiveness in this process. Future applications of this approach to update the priority areas might well involve richer data analysis and more extensive feedback from the public and health professionals.

Apply Improvability and Inclusiveness, Criteria

The recommendation to apply the improvability criterion after the impact criterion does not reflect the former's secondary status, but the fact that there was far less evidence available on improvability, and existing data could not easily be used for making comparisons across conditions. Therefore, the improvability criterion should be applied to high-impact areas to ensure that they can be improved within the current health system, and that evidence exists for believing that transforming the health system in these areas could result in widespread improvement for patients. Areas might be screened out at this step if they posed a large burden but were not improvable through interventions implemented within the health system. Finally, at each stage of the process, the list should be examined to ensure that it is inclusive across a range of populations, conditions, and quality improvement strategies.

Identify Priority Areas

The priority areas on the final list share a common set of features. The inclusion of each individual area is based on evidence of the need for improvement and of the likelihood that current treatments, if applied more effectively, would substantially enhance health. Collectively, the areas encompass all age groups and types of care (preventive, acute, chronic, and palliative) and represent a range of sectors of the health care system (hospitals, ambulatory care, home health). The list of candidates that emerges after all the criteria have been systematically applied should be carefully reassessed to ensure, to the extent possible, that all the criteria have been adequately met.

Implement Strategies for Improving Care, Measure Impact, and Review/Update List of Areas

Once the set of priority areas has been identified, steps should be taken to prepare for follow-up. Doing so will first and foremost require the development of national strategies for improving care within each of the priority areas. Next, it will be necessary to implement those strategies and measure their impact using methods that are standardized and permit comparison across the diverse areas of quality improvement involved. This assessment must include measures of the degree to which the system has been transformed and of the clinical impact on patient care.

As such changes are effected, the list of priority areas should be reviewed and updated—optimally every 3 to 5 years. Other areas may need to be added to the list as the result of new data on impact or the development of new treatment strategies. Likewise, if strategies for improvement are effective, it may be possible to remove some areas from the list.

> **Recommendation 4: The committee recommends that AHRQ, in collaboration with other private and public organizations, be responsible for continuous assessment of progress and updating of the list of priority areas. These responsibilities should include:**

- **Developing and improving data collection and measurement systems for assessing the effectiveness of quality improvement efforts.**

- **Supporting the development and dissemination of valid, accurate, and reliable standardized measures of quality.**

- **Measuring key attributes and outcomes and making this information available to the public.**

- **Revising the selection criteria and the list of priority areas.**

- **Reviewing the evidence base and results, and deciding on updated priorities every 3 to 5 years.**

- **Assessing changes in the attributes of society that affect health and health care and could alter the priority of various areas.**

- **Disseminating the results of strategies for quality improvement in the priority areas.**

Recommendation 5: The Committee recommends that data collection in the priority areas:

- **Go beyond the usual reliance on disease-and procedure-based information to include data on the health and functioning of the U.S. population.**

- **Cover relevant demographic and regional groups as well as the population as a whole, with particular emphasis on identifying disparities in care.**

- **Be consistent within and across categories to ensure accurate assessment and comparison of quality enhancement efforts.**

Recommendation 6: The committee recommends that the Congress and the Administration provide the necessary support for the ongoing process of monitoring progress in the priority areas and updating the list of areas. This support shall encompass:

- The administrative costs borne by AHRQ.

- The costs of developing and implementing data collection mechanisms and improving the capacity to measure results.

- The costs of investing strategically in research aimed at developing new scientific evidence on interventions that improve the quality of care and at creating additional accurate, valid, and reliable standardized measures of quality. Such research is especially critical in areas of high importance in which either the scientific evidence for effective interventions is lacking, or current measures of quality are inadequate.

Discussion of Limitations

The model recommended by the committee should not be viewed as a formal, structured, quantitative process, but as an interactive and qualitative approach to solving the complex problem under the committee's charge. It is too simplistic to think that a list of candidate priority areas could be screened through this step-by-step process to yield an unassailable final list. The committee struggled, for example, with how to balance the perceived need to make improvements in a particular area and a lack of evidence to support effective intervention at this point in time. There was debate over whether to focus on broader areas, such as heart disease, or narrower ones, such as hypertension. Some committee members believed that having a small number of priority areas might allow greater results within each area and facilitate the implementation of

effective interventions. However, others believed that a small number of conditions might exclude the involvement of some health professionals and fail to meet the need for equity and breadth. In the end, the committee decided to lean toward a larger number of priority areas.

In trying to strike a balance between including too many and too few areas, the committee reached consensus that to achieve inclusiveness, it would recommend 20 areas, but it would select within most of these areas a specific focus that would be expected to yield both large and achievable benefits. In most but not all instances, this focus was placed on interventions designed to prevent or retard the progression of early disease or risk factors. Thus, for example, while the area of diabetes is very broad, the committee is recommending a special focus on aggressive treatment and control of the disease in its early stages, given the strong evidence that such early treatment can substantially delay or prevent later complications. As noted elsewhere in the report, however, a number of areas believed to be important in terms of impact were not included in the final list because of a lack of scientific evidence of improvability or the absence of valid, reliable, and widely available measures.

The committee also recognizes the obvious limitation of having a relatively small number of individuals engaged in its deliberations. Although a concerted effort was made to have diverse groups represented among the committee members, it was impossible to include all stakeholders. The committee also faced considerable time constraints. Nonetheless, the committee believes that due consideration was given to a wide array of candidate priority areas and input received from a broad range of researchers and interest groups. The committee's recommended future process for priority setting would help address the limitations encountered during this study.

References

Centers for Disease Control and Prevention. 2000. *Unrealized Prevention Opportunities: Reducing the Health and Economic Burden of Chronic Disease.* Atlanta, GA: CDC, National Center for Chronic Disease Prevention and Health Promotion.

———. 2002. *The Burden of Chronic Diseases and Their Risk Factors.* Atlanta, GA: CDC, National Center for Chronic Disease Prevention and Health Promotion.

Cohen, S. B. 2001. Enhancements to the Medical Expenditure Panel Survey to improve health care expenditure and quality measurement. In Proceedings of the Statistics in Epidemiology Section, American Statistical Association.

———. 2002. *MEPS Enhancements to Support Healthcare Quality Measurements.* Presented at April 1-2, 2002 Priority Areas for Quality Improvement Meeting.

Daniels, N. 2000. Accountability for reasonableness. *BMJ* 321 (7272):1300-1.

Daniels, N., and J. Sabin. 1998. The ethics of accountability in managed care reform. *Health Aff (Millwood)* 17 (5):50-64.

Demakis, J. G., L. McQueen, K. W. Kizer, and J. R. Feussner. 2000. Quality Enhancement Research Initiative (QUERI): A collaboration between research and clinical practice. *Med Care* 38 (6 Suppl 1):I17-25 .

Feussner, J. R., K. W. Kizer, and J. G. Demakis. 2000. The Quality Enhancement Research Initiative (QUERI): From evidence to action. *Med Care* 38 (6 Suppl 1):I1-6.

Health Disparities Collaboratives. 2002. "Health Disparities Collaboratives." Online. Available at http://www.healthdisparities.net/ [accessed June 4, 2002].

Kizer, K. W., J. G. Demakis, and J. R. Feussner. 2000. Reinventing VA health care: Systematizing quality improvement and quality innovation. *Med Care* 38 (6 Suppl 1):I7-16.

Medical Expenditure Panel Survey. 2002. "Introduction to MEPS Data and Publications." Online. Available at http://www.meps.ahcpr. gov/Data_Public.htm [accessed June 4, 2002].

Michaud, C. M., C. J. Murray, and B. R. Bloom. 2001. Burden of disease: Implications for future research. *JAMA* 285 (5):535-9.

Murray, C. J., and A. D. Lopez. 1996. Evidence-based health policy: Lessons from the Global Burden of Disease Study. *Science* 274 (5288):740-3.

National Committee for Quality Assurance. 2002. *State of Health Care Quality Report.* Washington, DC: NCQA.

National Institutes of Health (NIH). 1997. "Setting Research Priorities at the National Institutes of Health." Online. Available at http://www.nih. gov/news/ResPriority/priority.htm [accessed June 4, 2002].

Partnership for Prevention. 2002. *Prevention Priorities: A Health Plan's Guide to the Highest Value Preventive Health Services.*

Stevens, D. M. 2002. *Changing Practice/Changing Lives.* Presented at May 9-10, 2002 Priority Areas for Quality Improvement Meeting.

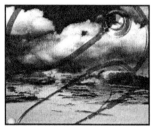 # Appendix A
Biographies of Committee Members

George J. Isham, MD, Chair

Dr. Isham is Medical Director and Chief Health Officer for HealthPartners. He is responsible for Quality and Utilization Management, chairs the Benefits Committee, and leads Partners for Better Health, a program and strategy for improving member health. Before assuming his current position, Dr. Isham was Medical Director of MedCenters Health Plan in Minneapolis. In the late 1980s, he was Executive Director of University Health Care, an organization affiliated with the University of Wisconsin in Madison. Dr. Isham received his master of science degree in preventive medicine/ administrative medicine at the University of Wisconsin Madison; he received his doctor of medicine degree from the University of Illinois; and he served his internship and residency in internal medicine at the University of Wisconsin Hospital and Clinics in Madison. Dr. Isham's practice experience as a primary care physician included 8 years at the Freeport Clinic in Freeport, Illinois, and more than 3 years as Clinical Assistant Professor in Medicine at the University of Wisconsin. HealthPartners is a consumer-governed Minnesota health plan. Formed through the 1992 affiliation of Group Health, Inc., and MedCenters Health Plan. HealthPartners is a large managed health care organization in Minnesota, representing nearly 800,000 members. Group Health, founded in 1957, is a network of staff medical and dental centers located throughout the Twin Cities. MedCenters, founded in 1972, is a network of contracted physicians serving members through affiliated medical and dental centers.

Brian Austin

Brian Austin is Deputy Director of Improving Chronic Illness Care, and as such has responsibility for overall administrative leadership of the program. He is Manager of the MacColl Institute for Healthcare Innovation, which he helped found in 1992. The MacColl Institute is devoted to developing, testing and disseminating innovations in the delivery of healthcare and is housed within Group Health Cooperative's Center for Health Studies in Seattle. Mr. Austin also serves on the administrative leadership team for the Center, a 200 person health services research department whose mission is to create and disseminate public-domain information regarding prevention and treatment of major health problems. He is active in all aspects of ICIC and the MacColl Institute, with special interest in incorporating new technologies into the primary care setting and the development of expert systems and improved practice team communication methods to enhance care delivery.

Stephen Berman, M.D.

Dr. Berman, a practicing primary care pediatrician, is a leader in child advocacy and health policy, a clinical researcher, and an educator. He is a Professor of Pediatrics and directs the Academic Section of General Pediatrics at the University of Colorado Health Sciences Center. He also served as past-President of the American Academy of Pediatrics. His commitment to clinical practice resulted in writing a textbook entitled *Pediatric Decision Making*. Dr. Berman has authored six child health bills enacted by his state legislature. These laws provide health insurance to low-income children; require seat belt use, and mandate immunizations and preventive care in insurance plans. He has developed several successful community service projects including the Reach Out project (funded by the RWJ foundation) to increase the participation of physicians in private practice in programs that serve low income underserved children, the Mile High Healthy Beginnings project (funded by both national and local foundations) to provide medical services to children enrolled in subsidized child care centers, and the Bright Beginnings project (funded by the Carnegie Foundation and local foundations) to provide volunteer home visits for families of newborns.

Karen A. Bodenhorn, RN, MPH

Karen A. Bodenhorn, RN, MPH, is President and CEO of the Center for Health Improvement (CHI), an independent, non-partisan, prevention-focused health policy and consulting center. CHI was founded with the mission to protect and improve the health of all Californians and has since established an impressive record for developing timely, user-friendly health policy documents, convening legislators and policy advocates to address health policy issues, and providing hands-on technical assistance to widely divergent groups within the healthcare community. Prior to launching CHI, Ms. Bodenhorn founded and directed Partnership for Prevention in Washington, D.C., a nonprofit organization created to increase national priority for prevention in health policy and practice. She also served as Vice President of Health Policy for a government relations consulting firm, representing a variety of clients before Congress and federal agencies. Ms. Bodenhorn earned her Master's Degree in Public Health from the University of North Carolina and her Bachelor of Science in Nursing from Duke University.

David M. Cutler, Ph.D.

David M. Cutler is a professor in the Department of Economics at the Kennedy School of Government at Harvard University (1991-present). He is also a research associate at the National Bureau of Economic Research, specializing in aging, health care, public economics and productivity programs. During 1993, Dr. Cutler served as a senior staff economist at the Council of Economic Advisors and Director of the National Economic Council. His research examines the impact of medical care on the public sector, the value of medical innovation and how population health is changing over time. He is editor of the *Journal of Health Economics* and has edited two books: *The Changing Hospital Industry: Comparing Not-for-Profit and For-Profit Hospitals* and *Medical Care Productivity and Output*. A member of the National Academy of Sciences, he was inducted into the Institute of Medicine (IOM) in 2001. He has served on two IOM Committees: the Committee on Future Directions in Behavioral and Social Sciences Research at NIH and the Committee on the NIH [National Institutes of Health] Research Priority-Setting Process.

Jaime A. Davidson, MD, FACP, FACE

Jaime A. Davidson is currently with Endocrine and Diabetes Associates of Texas, and is an Associate Professor of Medicine at the University of Texas, Southwestern Medical School. He is a regent for Midwestern State University, by appointment of the former Governor of Texas, George W. Bush. He serves as chair for the Managed Care Report Card of the Texas Diabetes Council, Texas Department of Health. He is also an advisor to the Food and Drug Administration for endocrinology and metabolic diseases. Dr. Davidson is serving a second term on the board of directors of the American Association of Clinical Endocrinologists, as well as the American College of Endocrinology. In the past he served as chair of the Texas Diabetes Council, Texas

Department of Health as well as on the National Diabetes Advisory Board at NIH; the Technical Advisory Committee, Centers for Disease Control (CDC); the Translation Committee and Latino Advisory Group to CDC for which he served as chair. He also served on the board of directors of the American Diabetes Association, and was chair of the Minority Committee and of "Diabetes Awareness and Resources for U.S. Latinos." He is past President of the American Diabetes Association, Texas Affiliate, and past President of the Endocrinology and Diabetes Association in the Texas Medical Association. He presently serves on several editorial boards: *Medico, Endocrine Practice, Medicina y Cultura*, and *Revista de Nutricion y Metabolismo*. He has received numerous awards, most recently the Rainbow Award from the American Diabetes Association and the Order of the Eagle from the American Association of Clinical Endocrinologists.

Benjamin G. Druss, MD, MPH

After graduating medical school, Dr. Druss received postgraduate training in primary care medicine, psychiatry, and health services research. He has been on the faculty of the Yale School of Medicine since 1996. His work has focused on understanding and improving care at the primary care/mental health interface in the United States. This research has examined such issues as the work and general health costs of mental illness, the quality of mental health care, and the quality and outcomes of general medical services for people with serious mental disorders. Dr. Druss collaborated on a study, recently published in *Health Affairs* (November/ December 2001), that compared the national economic burden of five chronic health conditions. He is currently working on developing strategies for improving the linkages between research and mental health policy. He has collaborated with and consulted for a number of public and private agencies, including the National Institute of Mental Health, the Washington Business Group, the

National Center for Quality Assurance, The Robert Wood Johnson Foundation, and the American Psychiatric Association. He was the recipient of the 2000 American Psychiatric Association Early Career Health Services Research Award, the 2000 Association for Health Services Research Article-of-the-Year Award, and the 2001 Chairman's Award for Outstanding Performance from the Yale Department of Psychiatry.

Jack C. Ebeler, MPA

Jack Ebeler is President and Chief Executive Officer of the Alliance of Community Health Plans, a national alliance of leading health plans whose members serve more than 11 million Americans, with approximately 100,000 affiliated physicians. Previously, he was Senior Vice President and Director of the Health Care Group at The Robert Wood Johnson Foundation. In 1995 and 1996, he served in the U.S. Department of Health and Human Services as Deputy Assistant Secretary for Planning and Evaluation/Health and then as Acting Assistant Secretary for Planning and Evaluation. Prior to that time, he served as Principal at Health Policy Alternatives, Inc., a consulting firm specializing in developing health policy and strategy options for a wide range of national and state health care associations and organizations (1987–1995). Previously, he was Vice President at Group Health, Inc. (now HealthPartners), a managed care plan in Minnesota, leading various departments including marketing and sales, strategic planning, member services, and corporate services (1983–1987).

Lisa I. Iezzoni, MD

Dr. Iezzoni is Professor of Medicine at Harvard Medical School and Co-Director of Research, Division of General Medicine and Primary Care, Department of Medicine, Beth Israel Deaconess Medical Center. Her research interests include: using risk adjustment to predict clinical outcomes and resource consumption; using administrative and clinical data to evaluate outcomes and assess quality of care; and improving daily functioning and quality of life for people with disabilities, especially impaired mobility. She is a member of the National Academy of Sciences, elected to the IOM in 2000. She has also served on three IOM committees: the Committee on Multiple Sclerosis: Current Status and Strategies for the Future, the Institutional Review Board Committee and the Committee to Advise the National Library of Medicine on Information Center Services.

Charles B. Inlander

Charles B. Inlander is President of the nonprofit People's Medical Society. Since its founding in early 1983, Mr. Inlander has guided the People's Medical Society to its status as one the most influential consumer health advocacy organizations in the United States. Mr. Inlander is a faculty lecturer at the Yale University School of Medicine; an adjunct faculty member at the Chicago-Kent College of Law; and a Fellow of the Institute for Science, Law and Technology at the Illinois Institute of Technology. He is a health commentator on Public Radio International's *MARKETPLACE*, heard throughout the country on public radio stations. He is a founder of the Civil Justice Foundation and serves, or has served, on the board of directors of Consumers for Civil Justice, the National League for Nursing, the Pennsylvania League for Nursing, and the Lehigh Valley Business Conference on Health Care. He is on the advisory boards of the Citizen Advocacy Center, the Primary Care Management Association, the American Academy of Family Physicians, HealthMarket, and *Bottom Line/Personal Publications*. He was a columnist in *Nursing Economics* and a contributing editor for *Medical Self-Care* magazine. He has authored or coauthored more than 20 best-selling consumer health books. His articles regularly appear in such publications as *The New York Times, Glamour,* and *Boardroom.* Prior to joining the People's Medical Society, Mr. Inlander established a national reputation as an advocate for the rights of handicapped citizens.

Joanne Lynn, MD

Dr. Lynn is a geriatrician who has taken on the challenge of improving end-of-life care. She has worked extensively to generate awareness of this need in both the public and private arenas. She is currently Director of The RAND Center to Improve Care of the Dying, a multidisciplinary center for research and education aimed at improving the care of seriously ill persons. She is also President of Americans for Better Care of the Dying (ABCD), a nonprofit public interest organization that promotes public understanding and coalitions across organizations to improve end-of-life care. Dr. Lynn was Project Director of the President's Commission for the Study of Ethical Problems in Medicine and Biomedical and Behavioral Research and principal writer of that commission's book, *Deciding to Forego Life-Sustaining Treatment: A Report on the Ethical, Medical and Legal Issues in Treatment Decisions.* A member of the National Academy of Sciences, she was elected to the IOM in 1996. She has served on numerous IOM committees, including the Committee on Care at the End of Life and the Committee to Study the Social and Ethical Impact of Biomedicine.

C. Tracy Orleans, Ph.D.

Dr. Orleans is responsible for program development and evaluation in the areas of health and behavior, tobacco control, and chronic disease management as Senior Scientist at The Robert Wood Johnson Foundation. During 1995–1999, she served as convener for the foundation's Tobacco Working Group.

Since 1999 she has directed the foundation's new efforts to promote the adoption of healthy behaviors, with special emphasis on physical activity. She has developed and led or co-led several of the foundation's major national programs in these areas, including Smoke-Free Families: Innovations to Stop Smoking During and Beyond Pregnancy (1993–2003), Cutting Back: Managed Care Screening and Brief Intervention for Risky Drinking (1996–2002), Addressing Tobacco in Managed Care (1996-2003), The National Spit Tobacco Education Program (1996–2003), Bridging the Gap: Research Informing Practice for Healthy Youth Behavior (1997–2002), Improving Chronic Illness Care (1998–2003), Physical Activity Policy and Environmental Research Initiative (2000–2005), and Helping Young Smokers Quit (2001–2005). A clinical psychologist, she is currently an Adjunct Full Member of the Fox Chase Cancer Center in Philadelphia, Pennsylvania. She also serves as an Adjunct Professor in the Department of Psychiatry at the University of Medicine and Dentistry of New Jersey and as a member of the U.S. Preventive Services Task Force.

Greg Pawlson, MD, MPH

Dr. Pawlson became Executive Vice President of the National Committee for Quality Assurance (NCQA) on January 1, 2000. His areas of responsibility at NCQA include performance measurement development, research, analysis, state and federal contracts, and the corporate–foundation relationship. Prior to joining NCQA, Dr. Pawlson was at The George Washington University Medical Center as Senior Associate Vice President for Health Affairs. Previously, he had served as Chairman of the Department of Health Care Sciences (DHCS) and Director of the Institute for Health Policy, Outcomes and Human Values at The George Washington University. Dr. Pawlson's areas of policy and research interest have included health professions education, health policy, health care financing, and, more recently, quality measurement and reporting.

His clinical career in geriatrics included both providing direct patient care and serving as a medical director in several nursing homes in Washington, D.C. Within organized medicine, Dr. Pawlson served as Chairman of the Public Policy Committee and later as President and Chairman of the Board of the American Geriatrics Society. He also served as a member of the National Council of the Society for General Internal Medicine and as Chairman of the Council of Department Chairs of the Society of Teachers of Preventive Medicine.

Paul D. Stolley, MD, MPH

Dr. Stolley is Professor in the Department of Epidemiology and Preventive Medicine at the University of Maryland School of Medicine, where he served as Department Chair during 1991–1999. Dr. Stolley is an epidemiologist and internist who trained at CDC's Epidemic Intelligence Service and The Johns Hopkins School of Hygiene and Public Health, where he also joined the faculty in the Department of Epidemiology. He then founded and led the Clinical Epidemiology Center at the University of Pennsylvania, where he served as Herbert Rorer Professor of Medicine. He is a member of the National Academy of Sciences and the IOM, where he has served on numerous committees, most recently the Committee on Examination of the Evolving Science for Dietary Supplements. He was previously President of the American Epidemiological Association, the American College of Epidemiology, and the Society for Epidemiologic Research.

Eugene Washington, MD, M.Sc.

Dr. Washington is Professor and Chair of the Department of Obstetrics, Gynecology and Reproductive Sciences at the University of California, San Francisco (UCSF). He is Director of UCSF's Medical Effectiveness Research Center for Diverse Populations and is also Director of the UCSF/Stanford Evidence-Based Practice Center. During 1990–1995, he served as a member of the U.S. Preventive Services Task Force, Office of the Assistant Secretary of Health, Department of Health and Human Services. His research interests include the effectiveness of reproductive health services, prevention of diseases in women, and how to explain and eliminating racial/ethnic health disparities. He is a member of the National Academy of Sciences, elected in 1997 to the IOM. He has served on numerous committees, most recently the Committee for Behavior Change in the 21st Century: Improving the Health of Diverse Populations and the subcommittee on Creating an Environment for Quality in Health Care.

Kevin Weiss, MD, MPH, FACP

Dr. Weiss is Professor of Medicine and Director of the Center for Healthcare Studies at Northwestern University Medical School, Chicago, Illinois, and Director of the Midwest Center for Health Services and Policy Research at Hines VA [Veterans Administration] Hospital, Hines, Illinois. Prior to assuming his current joint positions at Northwestern and the VA, Dr. Weiss was Associate Professor of Internal Medicine at Rush Medical College and Director of the Center for Health Services Research at the Rush Primary Care Institute, Rush-Presbyterian-St. Luke's Medical Center Chicago, Illinois. Previously, he was Associate Professor of Health Care Sciences and Medicine at The George Washington University Medical Center in Washington, DC, and Research Fellow at the Center for Health Policy Research at the George Washington University. He has previously held positions at the National Center for Health Statistics at the CDC, and the National Institute of Allergy and Infectious Diseases at the NIH. He is also a former Robert Wood Johnson Generalist Physician Faculty Scholar. Dr. Weiss conducts collaborative epidemiological and health services research projects addressing quality and access to care through practice guideline development and guideline implementation, chronic care disease management, and outcomes measurement. He has served on an IOM subcommittee on Building the 21st Century Health System.

Gail Wilensky, Ph.D.

Dr. Wilensky serves as John M. Olin Senior Fellow at Project HOPE, where she analyzes and develops policies relating to health reform and to ongoing changes in the medical marketplace. She also serves as Co-Chair of the President's Task Force to Improve Health Care Delivery for Our Nation's Veterans, which addresses health care for both veterans and military retirees. Dr. Wilensky testifies frequently before congressional committees; acts as an advisor to members of Congress and other elected officials; and speaks nationally and internationally before professional, business, and consumer groups. From 1997 to 2001, she chaired the Medicare Payment Advisory Commission, which advises Congress on payment and other issues relating to Medicare, and from 1995 to 1997, she chaired the Physician Payment Review Commission. Previously, she served as Deputy Assistant to President Bush for Policy Development, advising him on health and welfare issues. Prior to that, she was Administrator of the Health Care Financing Administration, overseeing the Medicare and Medicaid programs. Dr. Wilensky is an elected member of the IOM and its Governing Council, and serves as a trustee of the Combined Benefits Fund of the United Mineworkers of America and the Research Triangle Institute. She is an advisor to The Robert Wood Johnson Foundation and the Commonwealth Fund and is a director on several corporate boards. Dr. Wilensky received a bachelor's degree in psychology and a Ph.D. in economics at the University of Michigan.

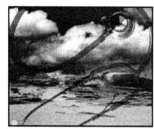# Appendix B
Committee on Identifying Priority Areas for Quality Improvement Workshop

WORKSHOP AGENDA

May 9–10, 2002

Holiday Inn Georgetown—Mirage Ballroom
2101 Wisconsin Ave., Washington, D.C.

MAY 9, 2002

Open Session

8:00–8:30 am	Continental Breakfast
8:30–8:45 am	**Welcome and Introductions**
	Overview of Workshop Goals
	George J. Isham, Committee Chair
8:45–9:15 am	**Panel #1: "Transformers" in Health Care—Integrated Delivery Models**
	Brian Austin Macoll Institute for Health Care Innovation
	David Stevens Health Resources and Services Administration

9:15–9:45 am	**Panel #2: "Transformers" in Health Care—Moving Towards Solutions**	
	Nico Pronk	HealthPartners
	Mary Tinetti	Yale School of Medicine

| 9:45–10:15 am | **Question and Answer Session for Panel 1 and 2 Presenters** |

| 10:15–10:30 am | Break |

10:30–11:00 am	**Panel #3: Health Burden and Costs of Various Conditions**	
	Benjamin Druss	Yale School of Medicine
	Gerard Anderson	The Johns Hopkins School of Public Health

| 11:00 – 11:30 am | **Question and Answer Session for Panel 3 Presenters** |

11:30 – 1:00 pm	**Luncheon Discussion**
	Priority Setting in Health Care: Philosophical Underpinnings
	Dan Brock	Brown University

1:00 - 2:15 pm	**Panel #4: Other Priority Areas Warranting Consideration**	
	Joanne Lynn	The RAND Corporation
		(end of life)
	Charlene Harrington	University of California - San Francisco
		(long term care)
	Bob Kafka	American Disabled for Accessible Public Transit
		(disability)
	Ken Wells	University of California, Los Angeles
		(mental health)
	James Perrin	Harvard Medical School
		(child/adolescent health)

| 2:15 – 3:15 pm | **Roundtable Discussion with Panel 4** |

| 3:15 – 3:30 pm | **Break** |

Closed Session

    3:30 - 5:30 pm   **Committee Deliberations on Criteria for Priority Areas**

MAY 10, 2002

Open Session

    8:00 – 8:30 am   Continental Breakfast

    8:30 – 8:45 am   **Welcome and Introductions**
                                Overview of Workshop Goals
                                  George J. Isham, Committee Chair

    8:45 –9:30 am   **Panel #5: Priority Setting for Preventive Services**

Ashley Coffield	Partnership for Prevention
Michael Maciosek	HealthPartners
Ali Mokdad	Centers for Disease Control and Prevention

    9:30 – 9:45 am   **Question and Answer Session for Panel 5 Presenters**

    9:45 – 10:00 am   **Break**

    10:00 – 10:45 am   **Panel # 6: Perspectives from the Business Community**

Helen Darling	Washington Business Group on Health
Suzanne Delbanco	Leapfrog Group
Kip Piper	National Health Care Purchasing Institute

    10:45 – 11:15 am   **Question and Answer Session for Panel 6 Presenters**

    11:15 – 12:00 noon   **Public Testimony**

Closed Session

    12:00 – 4:30 pm   **Working Lunch and Committee Deliberations on Criteria for Priority Areas**

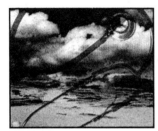

Appendix C
Priority Setting Models

Agency for Healthcare Research and Quality (AHRQ): Medical Expenditure Panel Survey

The Medical Expenditure Panel Survey (MEPS) provides national and regional annual estimates of health care utilization, expenditures, sources of payment, and insurance coverage for the U.S. noninstitutionalized population. AHRQ and the National Center for Heath Statistics cosponsor this initiative. MEPS comprises four survey components: the Household Component (HC), the Medical Provider Component (MPC), the Insurance Component, and the Nursing Home Component. The MEPS HC collects data on health conditions both at an individual and a household level. Other data drawn from this survey include demographics, health status, use of medical care services, charges and payments, access to care, satisfaction with care, health insurance coverage, income, and employment. Medical providers are contacted using the MEPS MPC to augment and verify the self-reported medical care events obtained from the MEPS HC (Medical Expenditure Panel Survey, 2002).

In planning for the MEPS health care quality enhancements, it was decided that a set of medical conditions would need to receive heightened attention. As a result, expansion of the HC was necessary to include individuals with illnesses that were of national concern. To facilitate the decision-making process or the selection of these conditions, the following criteria were established (Cohen, 2001):

- Prevalence—national prevalence rate for the medical condition (at least 3%)

- Availability of standardized questions used in other national surveys

- Accuracy of conditions households could report

- Availability of evidence-based quality measures

- Burden to society in terms of expenditures

Using these criteria, the following medical conditions were targeted by the MEPS healthcare quality enhancement effort: diabetes, asthma, hypertension, ischemic heart disease, arthritis, stroke, and chronic obstructive pulmonary disease.

Veterans Administration (VA): Quality Enhancement Research Initiative (QUERI)

QUERI is an integrated quality improvement program in use at the VA. QUERI'S underlying goals are to identify best practices, to incorporate them into daily use, and to provide a feedback mechanism to ensure continuous quality improvement. QUERI functions to translate findings in the research setting into improved patient care and system redesign (Demakis et al., 2000; Feussner et al., 2000; Kizer et al., 2000). A six-step process is employed to ensure systematic adherence to quality improvement efforts:

1. Identify high-risk/volume diseases among veterans.

2. Identify best practices.

3. Define existing practice patterns and outcomes across the VA and current variation from best practices.

4. Identify and implement interventions to promote best practices.

5. Document that best practices improve outcomes.

6. Document that outcomes are associated with improved health-related quality of life.

Eight targeted conditions were selected as the focal point for QUERI: chronic heart failure, diabetes, HIV/AIDS, ischemic heart disease, mental health (depression and schizophrenia),

spinal chord injury, and stroke. Criteria used to determine this group of conditions included the number of veterans affected, the burden of illness, and known health risks within the veteran population.

The Bureau of Primary Health Care/ Health Resources and Services Administration (HRSA/BPHC) Health Disparities Collaboratives

BPHC, part of HRSA within the Department of Health and Human Services (DHHS), provides funding for programs that expand access to high-quality, culturally and linguistically competent health care—both primary and preventive—for underserved, uninsured, and underinsured Americans. In 1998, BPHC organized five regional clusters of states and then funded one primary care association/clinical network team in each of these five clusters, along with the national clinical networks focused on oral health, migrant farm worker health care, and homeless health care (Health Disparities Collaboratives, 2002). These organizations then worked with the Institute for Healthcare Improvement (IHI) to develop the infrastructure for the Health Disparities Collaboratives.

The intent of these collaboratives is to change primary health care practices in order to improve the care provided to everyone and eliminate health disparities. To meet this goal, it was determined that the collaboratives should focus on a subgroup of the entire population and then, if successful, spread to the rest of the patients in a community.

The first collaborative, initiated in January 2000, focused on diabetes; it was quickly followed by the asthma and depression collaborative in March 2000. The program then expanded to cardiovascular disease in April 2001: future collaboratives are expected to include cancer, prevention, infant mortality, and immunizations (Health Disparities Collaboratives, 2002; Stevens, 2002).

Centers for Medicare and Medicaid Services (CMS)

CMS manages a national network of contractors known as quality improvement organizations (QIOs; formerly known as peer review organizations or PROs). The purpose of these QIOs is to systematically improve the quality of care received by Medicare beneficiaries in participating hospitals and now in an expanding group of providers in nonhospital settings. To provide guidance to the QIOs, CMS' Quality Improvement Program conducts an involved process to identify priority topic areas (Schulke, 2002). This process uses seven main criteria to assess the significance of proposed topics:

- Importance to Medicare population—How many people have the condition or receive the service? How many associated disabilities and/or deaths are associated with it?

- Science—Are there treatments that make a difference and measurements of their success?

- Performance gap—Does a gap exist between actual performance and what is achievable that results in substantial harm to the health of Medicare beneficiaries?

- Interventions—Are there interventions that QIOs can undertake to reduce the performance gap?

- Partnerships—Are there outside partners interested in this priority area that can contribute to its improvement? Are there internal department priorities that may make a topic more appealing?

- Cost—Can the cost to QIOs, providers, practitioners, and plans be reduced by focusing on this condition? Will the project increase or reduce Medicare trust fund outlays?

- Applicability to nonhospital settings

CMS applied these criteria to 31 proposed clinical topics that were listed for field implementation by QIOs in the Seventh QIO Statement of Work (Centers for Medicare and Medicade Services, 2002). Based on this assessment, CMS ultimately instructed the QIOs to focus on reducing clinical system failures for six priority topics: acute myocardial infarction, heart failure, pneumonia, postoperative infections, diabetes, and breast cancer.

Partnership for Prevention

The Partnership for Prevention, a national nonprofit organization supported by both the Centers for Disease Control and Prevention (CDC) and CMS, convened the Committee on Clinical Preventive Service Priorities to undertake the following two tasks: develop an approach for comparing clinical preventive services based on their relative value to society, and rank services recommended by the U.S. Preventive Services Task Force (Coffield et al., 2001; Maciosek et al., 2001).

To carry out the first task, two criteria were selected by the committee for evaluating the relative value clinical preventive services: clinically preventable burden (CPB), the proportion of disease & injury prevented by the service if it were delivered to 100 percent of the population at the recommended intervals; and cost effectiveness (CE), the costs of prevention minus costs averted divided by the number of quality-adjusted life years saved. Each clinical preventive service was assigned a separate CPB and CE score. These two scores were then summed and subsequently used to rank the 30 services being evaluated.

The majority of the highest-ranking scores turned out to be screening services. Vaccine services, such as the childhood mumps, measles, rubella vaccine received the highest overall ranking. Counseling services, including tobacco cessation counseling for adults and antitobacco messages for children, also figured prominently.

Seven services were highlighted from this final ranking to assist decision makers in determining how to target spending of limited health care dollars in this area most judiciously.

These rankings were compared with the current delivery rates at the national level.

The following services ranked high on the scale and were delivered to less than 50 percent of their targeted populations nationally:

- Assess adults for tobacco use, and provide counseling.

- Screen for vision impairment among adults older than age 65.

- Assess adolescents for drinking and drug use and provide counseling on abstinence

- Screen for colorectal cancer among persons older than age 50.

- Screen for chlamydia among women aged 15–24.

- Screen for problem drinking among adults, and provide counseling.

- Vaccinate adults older than age 65 against pneumococcal disease.

National Institutes of Health (NIH)

In response to pressure from advocacy groups and other stakeholders in biomedical science research, the NIH formed a working group to address priority setting for funding extramural research. Subsequently, Congress requested the Institute of Medicine (IOM) to review the priority setting process and criteria employed by NIH; the latter included public health needs, scientific quality of the research, probability of success, maintenance of a diverse portfolio, and maintenance of an adequate scientific infrastructure. Although the IOM supported the criteria chosen, recommendations for improvement were made. These included NIH increasing its use of health data, such data on disease as burden and cost, and gathering more input from the public (Gross et al., 1999).

NIH considers the following criteria for measuring health needs:

- Number of people with the disease (prevalence)

- Number of deaths caused by the disease

- Degree of disability caused by the disease

- Degree to which the disease shortens a normal productive lifetime

- Economic and social costs of the disease

- Need to respond rapidly to control the spread of a disease

NIH affirms that there are limitations to relying solely on any one of the mentioned criteria. Individually, they often lead to unintended outcomes. For example, if prevalence of disease were the dominant criteria, common diseases such as the common cold would receive the most attention. However, this approach could depress research on childhood cancers. Another case in point is mortality. By focusing on number of deaths, one may overlook chronic diseases, the very area on which the committee is focusing for efforts to restructure health care delivery restructuring efforts (National Institutes of Health (NIH), 1997).

References

Centers for Medicare and Medicade Services. 2002. "Quality Improvement Organizations (QIOs)." Online. Available at http://cms.hhs.gov/qio/2.asp [accessed Oct. 15, 2002].

Coffield, A. B., M. V. Maciosek, J. M. McGinnis, J. R. Harris, M. B. Caldwell, S. M. Teutsch, D. Atkins, J. H. Richland, and A. Haddix. 2001. Priorities among recommended clinical preventive services. *Am J Prev Med* 21 (1):1-9.

Cohen, S. B. 2001. Enhancements to the Medical Expenditure Panel Survey to improve health care expenditure and quality measurement. In Proceedings of the Statistics in Epidemiology Section, American Statistical Association.

Demakis, J. G., L. McQueen, K. W. Kizer, and J. R. Feussner. 2000. Quality Enhancement Research Initiative (QUERI): A collaboration between research and clinical practice. *Med Care* 38 (6 Suppl 1):I17-25 .

Feussner, J. R., K. W. Kizer, and J. G. Demakis. 2000. The Quality Enhancement Research Initiative (QUERI): From evidence to action. *Med Care* 38 (6 Suppl 1):I1-6.

Gross, C. P., G. F. Anderson, and N. R. Powe. 1999. The relation between funding by the National Institutes of Health and the burden of disease. *N Engl J Med* 340 (24):1881-7.

Health Disparities Collaboratives. 2002. "Health Disparities Collaboratives." Online. Available at http://www.healthdisparities.net/ [accessed June 4, 2002].

Kizer, K. W., J. G. Demakis, and J. R. Feussner. 2000. Reinventing VA health care: Systematizing quality improvement and quality innovation. *Med Care* 38 (6 Suppl 1):I7-16.

Maciosek, M. V., A. B. Coffield, J. M. McGinnis, J. R. Harris, M. B. Caldwell, S. M. Teutsch, D. Atkins, J. H. Richland, and A. Haddix. 2001. Methods for priority setting among clinical preventive services. *Am J Prev Med* 21 (1):10-9.

Medical Expenditure Panel Survey. 2002. "Medical Expenditure Panel Survey Website." Online. Available at http://www.meps.ahcpr.gov [accessed July 1, 2002].

National Institutes of Health (NIH). 1997. "Setting Research Priorities at the National Institutes of Health." Online. Available at http://www.nih.gov/news/ResPriority/priority.htm [accessed June 4, 2002].

Schulke, David Executive Vice President (American Health Quality Association). 30 April 2002. Process for Designating National Priority Clinical Topics for Medicare's Quality Improvement Program (Letter). Personal communication to George Isham, Chair (IOM Priority Areas for Quality Improvement Committee).

Stevens, D. M. 2002. *Changing Practice/Changing Lives.* Presented at May 9-10, 2002 Priority Areas for Quality Improvement Meeting.